PARANASAL SINUSES

Edited by **Balwant Singh Gendeh**

Paranasal Sinuses
http://dx.doi.org/10.5772/66003
Edited by Balwant Singh Gendeh

Contributors

Abdulmalik Saad Alsaied, Seçil Aksoy, Kaan Orhan, Ulas Oz, Eng Ooi, Benjamin Stew, Gokhan Gocmen, Yaşar Özkan, Tang-Chuan Wang, Che-Lun Hsu

Published by InTech
Janeza Trdine 9, 51000 Rijeka, Croatia

Publishing Process Manager Dajana Pemac
Technical Editor SPi Global
Cover InTech Design team

First published June, 2017
Printed in Croatia
Legal deposit, Croatia: National and University Library in Zagreb

Additional hard copies can be obtained from orders@intechopen.com

Paranasal Sinuses, Edited by Balwant Singh Gendeh
p. cm.
Print ISBN 978-953-51-3239-4
Online ISBN 978-953-51-3240-0

For EU product safety concerns:
IN TECH d.o.o., Prolaz Marije Krucifikse Kozulić 3, 51000 Rijeka, Croatia,
info@intechopen.com or visit our website at intechopen.com.

Meet the editor

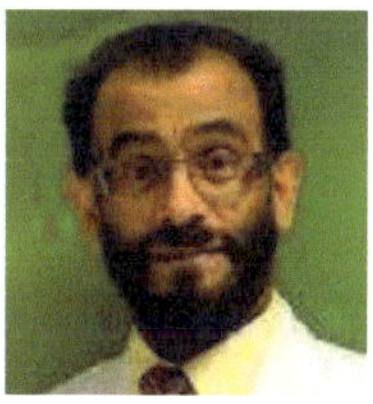

Dr. Balwant Singh Gendeh is a senior consultant ENT surgeon with sub-speciality interest in rhinology, namely, allergy, sinonasal diseases, endoscopic sinus, anterior and ventral skull base surgery and functional and cosmetic nasal surgery. He was a research registrar in ENT at the Royal Infirmary, Middlesbrough, United Kingdom, in 1993, and subsequently a JW Fulbright scholar at the University of Pittsburgh Medical Center (UPMC), Pittsburgh, USA, in 1997. During his Fulbright experience, he also worked at the Hospital of the University of Pennsylvania (HUP), Philadelphia, and St. Joseph's Hospital, Chicago, USA, sub-specializing in rhinology and aesthetic nasal surgery. Dr. BS Gendeh retired as a senior consultant ENT surgeon at the National University of Malaysia Medical Centre (UKMMC), presently is a visiting professor at the Department of Otorhinolaryngology-Head and Neck Surgery at UKMMC and is a resident ENT consultant at Pantai Hospital Kuala Lumpur since 2014. Due to his vast contribution to the academia in research and clinical publication, he was elected as a fellow of the Academy of Sciences Malaysia in April 2016.

Contents

Preface

This book covers selected topics in rhinology, providing a journey into advancements in various aspects of the field. A collection of manuscripts of this nature involves extensive exposure and accumulation of knowledge from experience collected over many years. The topics cover both basic and clinical concepts of rhinology. Each author contributed his/her own perspective on each topic adding theories, future trends and research findings.

The chapters of this book are arranged under five sections, namely, 'Surgical Anatomy', 'Dental-Related Diseases', 'Radiological Imaging', 'Nasal Spaces' and 'Surgical Training'. This book is intended for general otolaryngologists, sub-specialists, researches, residents and fellows. Therefore, it should encourage researchers and clinicians to innovate new ideas for future basic research and clinical practice.

The outcome of input from multi-national–related otolaryngologists/rhinologists from all over the world with a common goal towards better human health care has been collected in this book publication. Some of the authors are very experienced, while some are newcomers as researchers or clinicians.

This book is accessible online to allow free access to as many readers as possible. It is also available in print for those who do not have Internet access or are interested in having their own hard copy. This book will ultimately contribute to the global distribution of knowledge in rhinology between researchers and clinicians.

I would like to congratulate each and every one of the contributors for his/her excellent input on each chapter. Each author sacrificed his/her valuable time and effort to write a chapter resulting in the success of this book. I would like to thank Ms. Dajana Pemac, the publishing process manager, for her expert assistance on all issues concerning the book; Ms. Sandra Bakić, the commissioning editor, for her tireless assistance; and to all for choosing me to be the editor of this book. My kind gratitude goes to the technical editors for arranging the book in a uniform format and InTech Open Access Publisher for undertaking this novel mission. I hope that this book will be part of a series of books in all sub-specialities of rhinology and that it will enhance global collaboration not only between physicians but also for betterment of humankind. I wish the reader an enjoyable journey and hope you will find this book interesting.

I would like to thank my teachers and students from whom I gained knowledge throughout the years. Lastly, I dedicate this book to my wife Dr. Pritam Kaur Mangat, my daughter Dr. Manvin Kaur Gendeh, her husband Dr. Avinesh Singh Bhar and my son Dr. Hardip Singh Gendeh for all their patience and understanding.

Balwant Singh Gendeh,
MBBS (Kashmir), MS(ORL-HNS) UKM, AM (Mal), FAMM, FASc (M'sia)
Visiting Professor and Senior Consultant ENT Surgeon/Rhinologist
(Endoscopic Sinus/Skull Base Surgery and Functional and Cosmetic Nasal Surgery),
Department of Otorhinolaryngology-Head and Neck Surgery (ORL-HNS),
National University Malaysia Medical Centre (UKMMC),
Resident ENT Surgeon, Pantai Hospital
Kuala Lumpur, Malaysia

Section 1

Surgical Anatomy

Chapter 1

Paranasal Sinus Anatomy: What the Surgeon Needs to Know

Abdulmalik S. Alsaied

Additional information is available at the end of the chapter

http://dx.doi.org/10.5772/intechopen.69089

Abstract

Performing a smooth and clean sinus surgery goes hand in hand with a perfect understanding of the nasal and paranasal anatomy. Within this chapter, the paranasal and related structures surgical anatomy will be extensively reviewed, with emphasis on the anatomical landmarks and the normal anatomical variations, which have a significant impact on the function, pathology, and surgical procedures of the paranasal sinuses.

Keywords: paranasal sinuses, anatomy, maxillary, ethmoid, frontal, sphenoid, endoscopic sinus surgery

1. Introduction

The solid knowledge of the surgical anatomy and normal development of the paranasal sinuses is the key element behind achieving superb end results, whether the target is to accomplish a therapeutic surgical procedure or to conduct a clinical trial or research. Understanding the surgical landmarks and the anatomical variants of the paranasal sinuses will guide surgeons to a safe, uncomplicated, and successful endoscopic sinus surgery.

2. Histology of the nose and paranasal sinuses

The nasal cavity and all paranasal sinuses are lined by respiratory pseudostratified epithelium except areas of the roof of the cavity, most superior part of nasal septum, and the medial part of superior turbinate are lined by mucosa that contains receptors for the smell sensation known as olfactory area. On the lateral wall and within the sinuses, the mucosa is highly vascularized and adherent to the periosteum of the underlying bone.

Respiratory epithelium contains four types of cells:

1. **Columnar cells:** Divided into ciliated and non-ciliated. The anterior part of the nasal cavity has non-ciliated columnar cells, and the ciliated cells start from the head of inferior turbinate and posteriorly. Mucosa of the paranasal sinuses is high in the concentration of the ciliated columnar cells. Each ciliated cell contains around 100 cilia. Concentration of the ciliated cells varies within the nasal and paranasal mucosa. Giving the fact that cold, dry, and high airflow decreases the number of ciliated cells within the mucosa, which explains why the anterior nasal mucosa has less ciliated cells comparing with the posterior mucosa. And in cases of deviated nasal septum, the narrower sides have higher concentration of ciliated cells than the wider sides.
2. **Goblet cells:** The number of goblet cells varies within the nasal and sinuses mucosa, the posterior we go, the higher number of goblet cells we find. They are sensitive to mechanical and chemical stimulus; however, their contribution to nasal secretion is minimum.
3. **Basal cells:** They are the progenitors of the other type of cells. They are located deep on the basement membrane and not reaching the surface.
4. **Basement membrane:** The deepest layer of the epithelium, which consists of collagen fibrils. It became thicker in individuals with rhinitis [1].

3. Nasal cavity

Nasal cavity is divided by the nasal septum into two halves, so the septum forms the medial wall of these two nasal cavities. The lateral wall of each cavity contains three projections called turbinates or conchae (occasionally four turbinates) and contains passages under these turbinates as well. The roof formed by a sieve-like bone called cribriform plate of the ethmoid, which separates the nasal cavity from anterior cranial fossa. Olfactory nerves pierce through the cribriform plate on each side. Anteriorly, the roof is sloping downward in form of nasal spine of the frontal bone and nasal bone. Posteriorly, it is sloping downward as the face of sphenoid sinus. The floor of the nasal cavity, which is wider than the roof, is formed by the palatine process of the maxilla anteriorly and the horizontal process of the palatine bone posterior to it. In adult individual, the average surface area is about 150 cm^2 and the average volume is about 15 ml for both nasal cavities [1, 2].

3.1. Nasal septum

The nasal septum consists of three parts: (1) the cartilaginous septum (quadrangular cartilage), anteriorly; (2) the bony septum posteriorly, which comprises two bones (the upper one is the perpendicular plate of the ethmoid and the lower one is the vomer); (3) the membranous septum, which is the smallest and the most caudal part, is located between the quadrangular cartilage and the columella. It is not unusual to have a deviated septum toward either sides, making one side narrower than the other [3].

3.2. Lateral nasal wall

The lateral wall of the nasal cavity is a complex structure formed by the inferior, middle, and superior turbinates and, occasionally, the supreme turbinate, the fourth turbinate. Lateral to these turbinates are the corresponding meatuses. The paranasal sinuses are divided per their drainage systems into anterior sinuses group (maxillary, anterior ethmoid, and frontal sinuses) which drains into the middle meatus through the anterior ostiomeatal unit. And the posterior sinuses group (posterior ethmoid and sphenoid sinuses) drains into the sphenoethmoidal recess (aka posterior ostiomeatal unit) (**Figure 1**). The lateral wall also has the drainage of nasolacrimal apparatus via the nasolacrimal duct to the inferior meatus. In addition, it has the sphenopalatine foramen, which connects the nasal cavity to pterygopalatine fossa.

3.3. Turbinates and meatuses

3.3.1. Inferior turbinate and meatus

Unlike the superior and middle turbinates, which are parts of the ethmoid bone, the inferior turbinate is an independent bone. It is the largest one among them and it extends along the

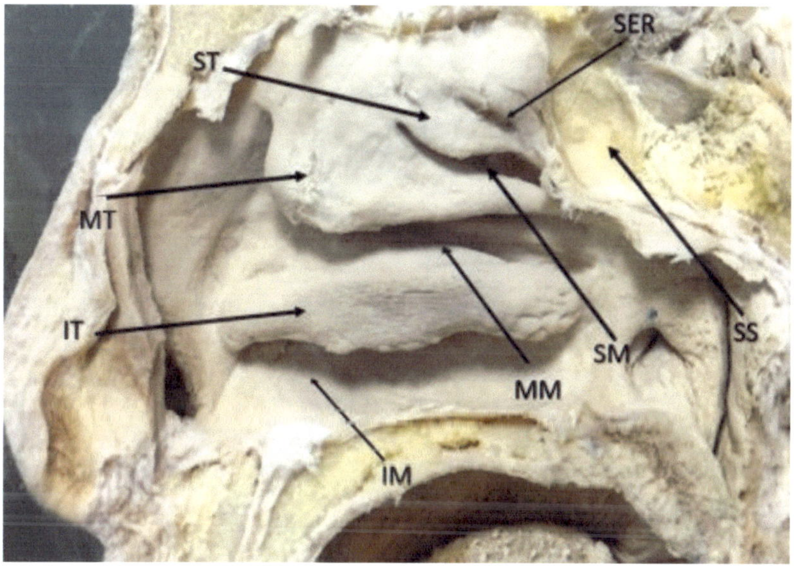

Figure 1. Gross picture of a parasagittal view of the lateral nasal wall. IT, inferior turbinate; MT, middle turbinate; ST, superior turbinate; IM, inferior meatus; MM, middle meatus; SM, superior meatus; SER, sphenoethmoidal recess; SS, sphenoid sinus.

entire length of the nasal floor. Anteriorly, it articulates with the conchal crest of the maxilla, the middle part of the turbinate covers the lower portion of the medial wall of maxillary sinus. Posteriorly, inferior turbinate articulates with the conchal crest of palatine bone. In the inferior meatus, the nasolacrimal duct opens about 2 cm behind the nostril.

3.3.2. Middle turbinate and meatus

The middle turbinate extends along the middle and posterior parts of the nasal cavity. It has three attachments which make it a very stable structure.

- Anterior attachment is vertically oriented and attached superiorly to the lateral border of cribriform plate.
- Second attachment is obliquely oriented, forming the basal lamella or "ground lamella" (which is the most important one in providing the stability of the middle turbinate); it is attached to the lamina papyracea (medial wall of the orbit).
- Posterior attachment is attached to the medial wall of maxillary sinus, and it is horizontally oriented.

The basal lamella divides the ethmoid sinus into anterior and posterior air cells. Immediately behind the posterior part of the middle turbinate underneath the mucosa is the sphenopalatine foramen. The middle meatus receives drainage of the anterior sinuses group as a component of the anterior ostiomeatal unit.

3.3.3. Superior turbinate and meatus

Superior turbinate occupies only the upper part of nasal cavity. Occasionally, there is a fourth turbinate called the supreme turbinate, and the corresponding meatus is the supreme meatus. The posterior ethmoid cells drain into the superior meatus. The supreme meatus "if present" drains the most posterior ethmoid cells.

3.3.4. Anatomical variations of the turbinates

- **Concha bullosa:** It is a pneumatization of the inferior bulbous part of middle turbinate. Occurs in approximately 24–55% of the population and often bilateral. Usually pneumatization originates from the frontal recess or the agger nasi cell [4, 5] (**Figure 2**).
- **Interlamellar cell of Grunwald:** Also called lamellar bulla or conchal neck air cell. It occurs when the pneumatization is limited to the vertical part of middle turbinate. Usually not causing narrowing of the ostiomeatal unit [6] (**Figure 3**).
- **Paradoxic middle turbinate:** Present in about 26% of the population. Occasionally, it can affect the patency of the ostiomeatal unit [6] (**Figure 4**).
- **Pneumatized basal lamella:** Can be falsely considered as a posterior ethmoid air cell during endoscopic sinus surgery.

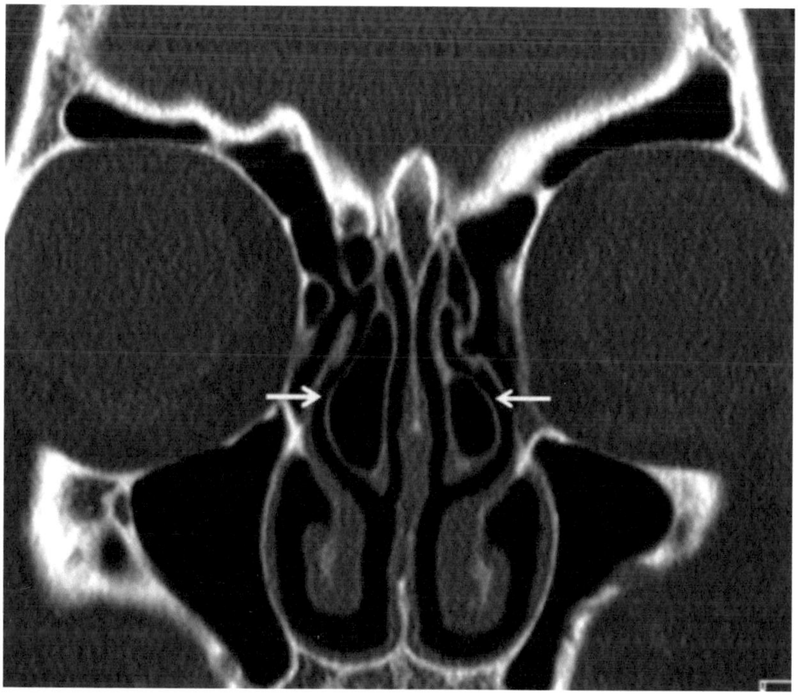

Figure 2. Coronal computed tomography "CT" scan showing pneumatization of the bulbous portion of middle turbinate bilaterally "concha bullosa" (arrows).

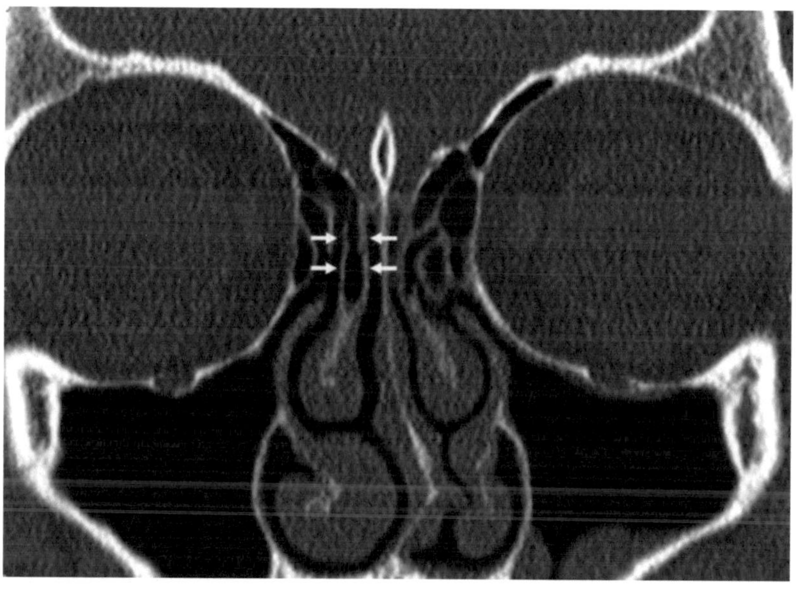

Figure 3. Coronal CT scan showing pneumatization that is restricted to the vertical lamella of the right middle turbinate "interlamellar cell of Grunwald" (arrows).

- **Missed basal lamella:** When the basal lamella does not attach to the lamina papyracea, it attaches to the lateral maxillary sinus wall.
- Rare variations like pneumatization of inferior turbinate, bifid inferior turbinate, and second middle turbinate have been reported in the literature [7–9].

3.4. Ostiomeatal unit

The anterior ostiomeatal unit drains the maxillary, anterior ethmoid, and frontal sinuses. It is formed by (1) ethmoid infundibulum, (2) middle meatus, (3) hiatus semilunaris, (4) maxillary ostium, (5) ethmoid bulla, (6) frontal recess, and (7) uncinate process (**Figure 5**). Occasionally, abnormalities or anatomical variations could affect the patency of this unit. The other draining ostiomeatal unit, located posterior in the nasal cavity, is the sphenoethmoidal recess. It drains the posterior ethmoid sinus lateral to the superior turbinate and drains the sphenoid sinus medial to the superior turbinate [6, 10].

3.4.1. Uncinate process

The uncinate process is a crescent-shaped, thin individual bone. Inferiorly, it is attached to the ethmoidal process of inferior turbinate. The anterior attachment of uncinate process is to the lacrimal bone. Posteriorly, uncinate process forms the anteroinferior border of the hiatus semilunaris. Medial to the uncinate is the ethmoid infundibulum, and laterally is the middle meatus. The superior attachment of the uncinate process is the most interesting one, that is, because of its variability and its direct effect on frontal sinus drainage pathway. There are three patterns of attachment of the superior portion of the uncinate:

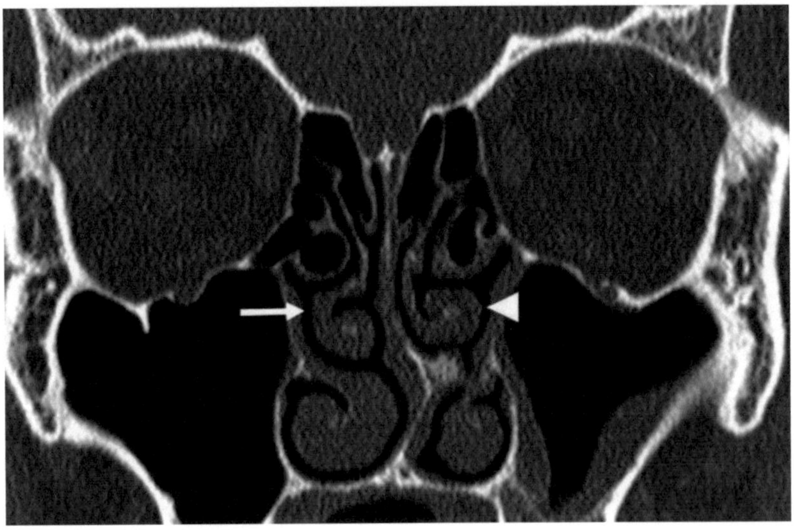

Figure 4. Coronal CT scan demonstrating paradoxical right middle turbinate (arrow). Left middle turbinate is indicated (arrowhead) for comparison, showing the normal orientation.

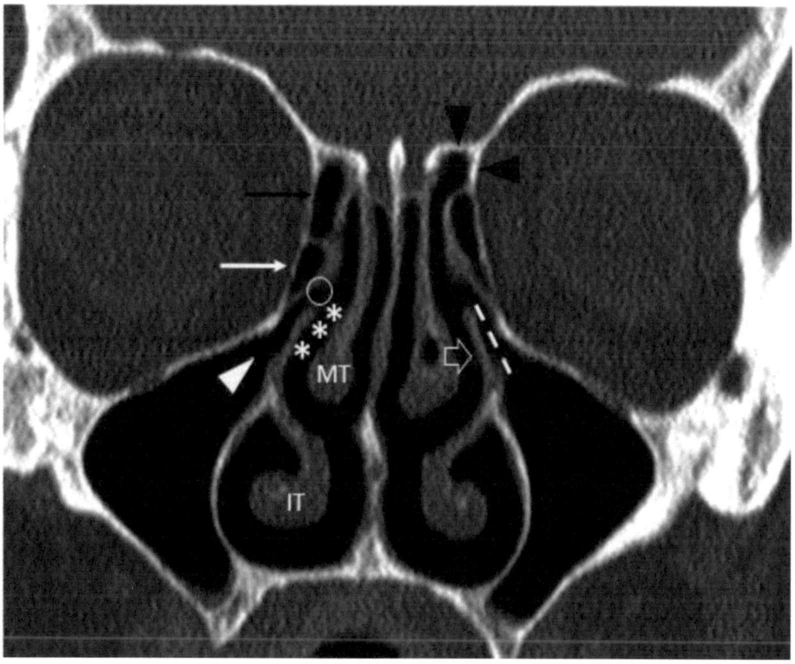

Figure 5. Coronal CT scan showing the components of the ostiomeatal unit: ethmoid bulla (white arrow); maxillary sinus ostium (white arrowhead), middle meatus (asterisks); uncinate process (hollow arrow); hiatus semilunaris "the space between the uncinate process and ethmoid bulla" (white circle); ethmoid infundibulum (dashed line). Frontal recess is part of the ostiomeatal unit (not shown in this coronal level, seen on more anterior view). Note the suprabullar recess on the left side (black arrowheads), which is the space created above the ethmoid bulla when the roof of bulla does not reach up to the skull base, superiorly. On the right side, suprabullar air cell (black arrow) "covered in later sections within this article." MT, middle turbinate; IT, inferior turbinate.

1. **Attachment to the lamina papyracea:** The most common site, found in about 50% of individuals. In this case, frontal sinus drainage pathway drains into the middle meatus. A lateral blind pouch will be formed between the uncinate and the lamina papyracea called the terminal recess or "recessus terminalis" (**Figure 6A**).

2. **Attachment to the middle turbinate:** The uncinate process displaced medially by the large agger nasi air cell and attached to the middle turbinate. Frontal sinus drains into the ethmoid infundibulum with this type (**Figure 6B**).

3. **Attachment to the skull base:** The least often site of attachment. The uncinate process extends superiorly to the skull base without contacting the agger nasi air cell. Here, frontal sinus drains into the ethmoid infundibulum as well (**Figure 6C**).

3.4.1.1. Anatomical variations of uncinate process

- **Pneumatized uncinate process (Uncinate bulla):** Literature reports a rate of about 0.4–2.5% of pneumatized uncinate process. If it is large enough, this could affect the patency of ostiomeatal unit [11, 12] (**Figure 7**).

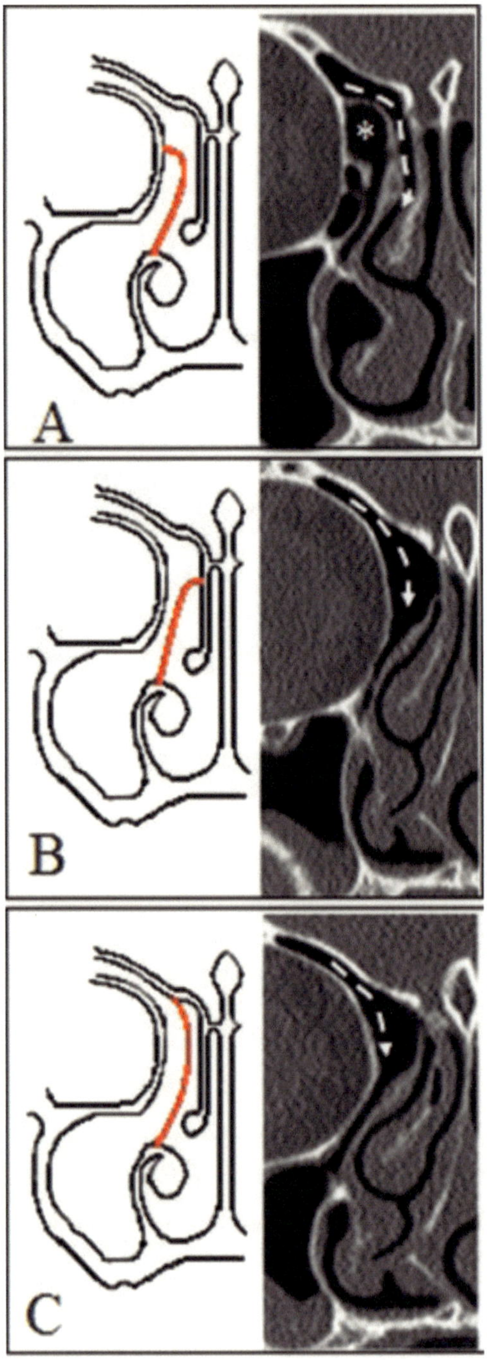

Figure 6. Variant attachments of the uncinate process (red). (A) Attachment to lamina papyracea. Note the blind pouch created between the uncinate and lamina papyracea "recess terminalis (asterisk)." Frontal sinus drains medial to the uncinate into the middle meatus (dashed arrow). (B) Attachment to middle turbinate. Frontal sinus drains into the ethmoid infundibulum. (C) Attachment to skull base. Also, the frontal sinus drainage pathway ends into the ethmoid infundibulum with this type.

http://dx.doi.org/10.5772/intechopen.69089

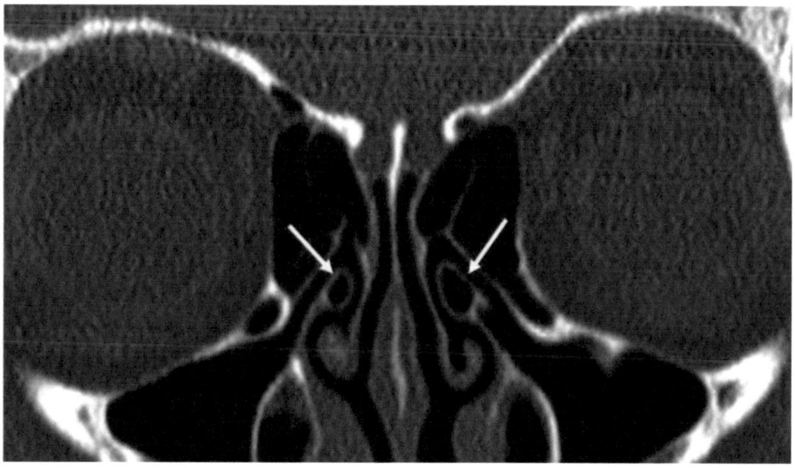

Figure 7. Coronal CT scan showing bilateral pneumatized uncinate process "uncinate bulla" (arrows). Note that ostio-meatal units are patent bilaterally; however, extensive pneumatization might compromise it.

- **Atelectatic uncinate process:** The uncinate will be adherent to the inferomedial wall of the orbit. Often seen in maxillary sinus hypoplasia or silent sinus syndrome. This condition increases the risk of inadvertent violation of the orbit during endoscopic sinus surgery.
- **Horizontal uncinate process:** Almost always associated with large ethmoid bulla. Rarely the uncinate process could be totally absent.

3.4.2. Hiatus semilunaris and ethmoid infundibulum

The space between the anterior wall of ethmoid bulla and the free edge of uncinate process is called the hiatus semilunaris; it opens anterosuperiorly into a cavity called the ethmoid infundibulum. The ethmoid infundibulum is the space between the uncinate process and the inferomedial wall of the orbit (**Figure 5**). Hiatus semilunaris receives drainage from the ethmoid bulla. The maxillary sinus and often the frontal sinus, depending on the superior attachment of the uncinate process, drain into the ethmoid infundibulum.

3.5. Olfactory fossa

The olfactory fossa contains olfactory bulbs and blood vessels. Its boundaries are inferiorly the cribriform plate of the ethmoid and medially the crista galli. Laterally it is bounded by the thinnest bone in the anterior skull base "the lateral lamella of the cribriform plate." Superiorly it communicates with the anterior cranial fossa.

Keros in 1962 classified the depth of olfactory fossa into three types based on the length of the lateral lamella [13]:

- **Type 1:** The length of the lateral lamella is 1–3 mm, suggesting a shallow olfactory fossa seen in 12% of the population.

- **Type 2:** The length of the lateral lamella is 4–7 mm, means a moderately deep olfactory fossa seen in 70% of the population.
- **Type 3:** The lateral lamella is longer, measuring 8–16 mm indicating a deep olfactory fossa seen in 18% of the population (**Figure 8**).

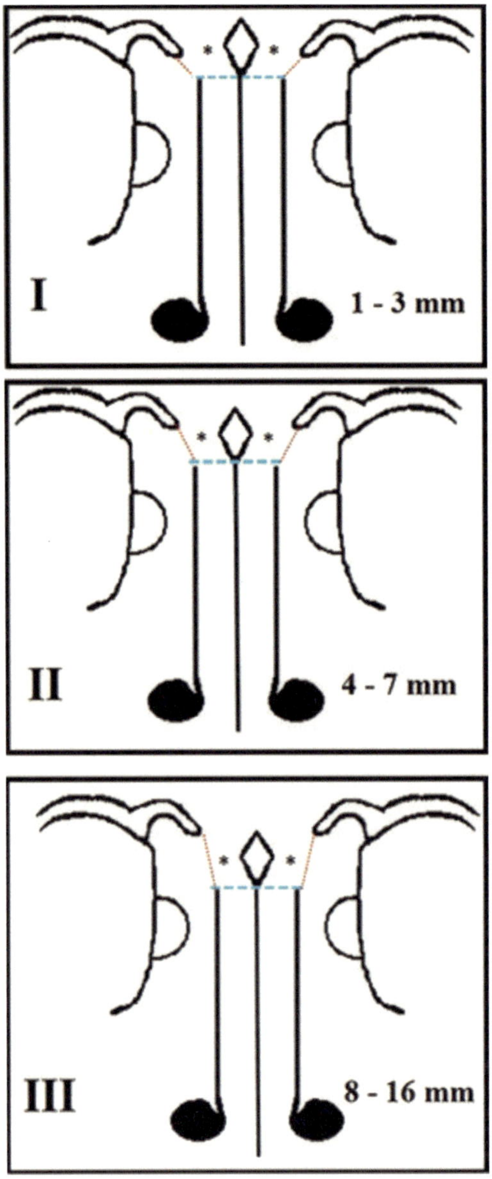

Figure 8. Coronal view of the olfactory fossa (asterisks) and its variations of depth. Thick dashed line represents the cribriform plate of the ethmoid. Thin dashed lines represent the thin lateral lamella of the cribriform. The depth of the olfactory fossa classified based on the length of the lateral lamella. Type I: lateral lamella length 1–3 mm; type II: lateral lamella length 4–7 mm; and type III: lateral lamella length 8–16 mm.

An anatomical variation of asymmetry in the depth of olfactory fossa had been reported in literature in up to 10–30% of the population [14].

Both type 1 and type 3 olfactory fossae are at increased risk for injury during endoscopic sinus surgery because in type 1 the angle between the medial and lateral lamellae of the cribriform plate is greater, and in type 3 the olfactory fossa is lower.

3.6. Blood supply, innervation, and lymphatic drainage of the nasal cavity

The nasal cavity is supplied by circulation derived from the internal and external carotid arteries, namely anterior and posterior ethmoidal arteries, sphenopalatine artery, septal branch of the superior labial artery, and the greater and ascending palatine arteries. Sphenopalatine artery is the main supplier of the nasal cavity.

In the lateral nasal wall, sphenopalatine artery after entering the nasal cavity through the sphenopalatine foramen gives off its posterior lateral nasal branches to supply the lateral wall. And it crosses the face of sphenoid sinus toward the posterior end of nasal septum as the posterior septal artery.

Veins accompany the arteries and drain to pterygoid plexus, facial vein, ophthalmic, and inferior cerebral veins [15].

Lateral nasal wall receives innervation from many nerves. Infraorbital nerves supply the vestibular area. The anterior ethmoidal nerve supplies the superior part of lateral wall. And the anterior superior alveolar nerve innervates the mucosa at the level of the wall of the maxillary sinus. The upper back mucosa is supplied by the lateral posterior superior nasal nerve. And the lower back mucosa innervated by the posterior inferior nasal nerve. The parasympathetic fibers reach the nasal cavity in the vidian nerve, and sympathetic fibers follow the blood vessels.

Lymphatic drainage of nasal cavity is to the submandibular, deep cervical, and retropharyngeal nodes.

4. Maxillary sinus

Maxillary sinus occupies the body of the maxillary bone. It is pyramidal in shape, with the base facing medially. The roof of the sinus is the orbital floor, and sinus's floor is formed by the alveolar process of the maxilla.

The medial wall of the maxilla is a large bony defect, known as "the fontanelle," in which the lateral nasal wall mucosa lies directly over the maxillary sinus medial wall mucosa. However, the bony defect is made much smaller by the contribution of the surrounding bones like lacrimal bone, ethmoid bone, inferior turbinate, and perpendicular plate of the palatine bone. This fontanelle is crossed by the uncinate process which divided it into a small anterior fontanelle and larger posterior fontanelle [16].

In adult individual, the maxillary sinus may extend from the area of the premolar teeth to the third molar, with a volume of approximately 15–22 ml [17].

In hyperpneumatized sinus, the apices of the molars or premolars are separated by a thin bone from the floor of the maxillary sinus or even project into the sinus floor. Occasionally, this bone is very thin or even absent, making extraction of such a tooth risky to leave a fistula by tearing of the mucous membrane. However, these types of fistulae often end with spontaneous healing [18].

Immediately posterior to the maxillary sinus lie the infratemporal fossa laterally and the pterygopalatine fossa medially.

4.1. Infraorbital nerve

The infraorbital nerve, a branch of the maxillary division "V2" of the trigeminal nerve, crosses the roof of maxillary sinus within a bony canal that opens as the infraorbital foramen, about 1 cm below the infraorbital rim (**Figure 9A**).

The inferior wall of the infraorbital canal can be extremely thin, with an average thickness of 0.2 mm or it may be completely dehiscent in between 12 and 16% of cases. It can be abnormally protruded within the maxillary sinus as well [19] (**Figures 9B** and **C** and **12**). In these situations, surgeon must identify these variants if present and pay extra attention during the procedure not to injure the nerve.

4.2. Maxillary sinus natural ostium

Ostium of the maxillary sinus is located in the upper portion of the medial wall of the sinus, and it opens at the posterior end of the hiatus semilunaris below the ethmoid bulla. The diameter of the ostium is about 2–4 mm, but it can be as wide as 10 mm. Mostly, the ostium existed as a canal with inferolateral orientation toward the sinus; however, it might be only an opening in some cases [20].

4.3. Development of maxillary sinus

Although the development of maxillary sinus starts in the intrauterine period, at birth it is not more than a shallow sac below the medial side of the orbital floor.

The growth of maxillary sinus is characterized by biphasic rapid growth, first phase during the first 3 years of life and the second phase from 7 to 12 years of age. A slow pneumatization continues until the age of 20 years as well.

- By the age of four, the lateral wall of the sinus reaches the infraorbital canal.
- By the age of seven, the floor reaches the level of inferior turbinate.
- By the age of nine, the floor of maxillary sinus reaches the level of the floor of nasal cavity.
- In adult individual, the floor of the sinus extends about 1 cm below the level of the floor of nasal cavity [21].

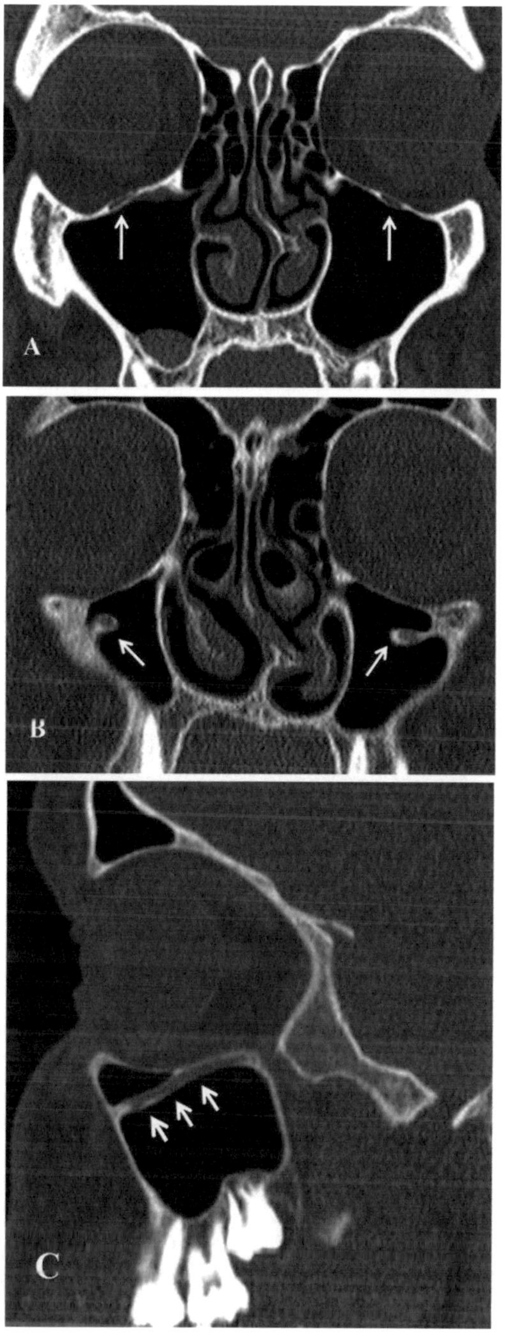

Figure 9. Coronal and sagittal CT scan. (A) Normal infraorbital bony canal (arrows) note the thin bony walls of the canal. (B) Bilateral aberrant locations of the infraorbital canals (arrows). They are protruded into the sinus which put the nerves at risk of traumatic injury during endoscopic maxillary sinus surgery. (C) Sagittal view for the left maxillary sinus of same patient in (B), demonstrating how the infraorbital canal is abnormally crossing the maxillary sinus (small arrows).

4.4. Anatomical variations of maxillary sinus

- **Accessory sinus ostium:** Any maxillary sinus opening outside the hiatus semilunaris is considered an accessory ostium. Its incidence is about 10–16%; however, some literature report a higher rate [22]. It is located in the posterior fontanelle, posterior to natural ostium (**Figure 10**). Typically, it is smaller than the natural ostium with an average diameter of 1.5 mm. The clinical significance of the presence of an accessory ostium is that occasionally a circular flow of mucus between the natural and the accessory ostia could occur, leading to recurrent sinusitis. If an accessory ostium is encountered intraoperatively, it should be surgically connected with the natural ostium.
- **Maxillary sinus hypoplasia:** It could be a genuine variant in about 10% of the population [4]. However, it might be secondary to other conditions like silent sinus syndrome, post-operated, or post-traumatic sinus. It carries a higher risk of orbital penetration during endoscopic sinus surgery.
- **Maxillary sinus septum:** Maxillary sinus septum is defined as a ridge that is 2.5 mm or more in height. It can be bony or fibrous septum [23]. Usually extends from the infraorbital canal to the lateral wall of the sinus. Occasionally it can impair the drainage of the sinus (**Figure 11**).
- **Infraorbital cell (Haller cell):** Any extension of the anterior ethmoid air cells along the orbital floor and lateral to the lamina papyracea is considered an infraorbital cell (**Figure 12**). The incidence of this variation ranges from 10 to 18% in the literature. It might compromise the patency of the maxillary ostium [24].

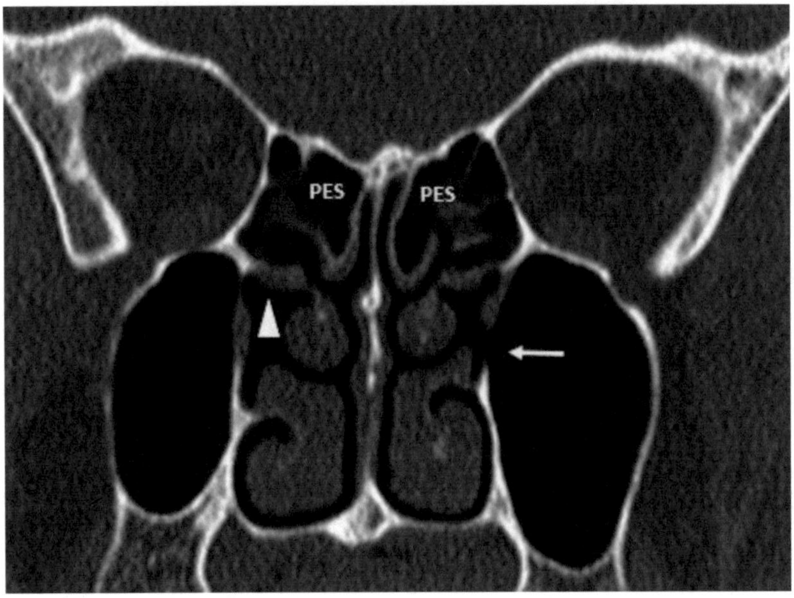

Figure 10. Coronal CT scan showing an accessory maxillary sinus ostium at the left maxillary sinus (arrow). It is located posterior to natural ostium, note the presence of the horizontal "third" part of middle turbinate (arrowhead), and the posterior ethmoid air cells (PES) indicate a posterior level of the view.

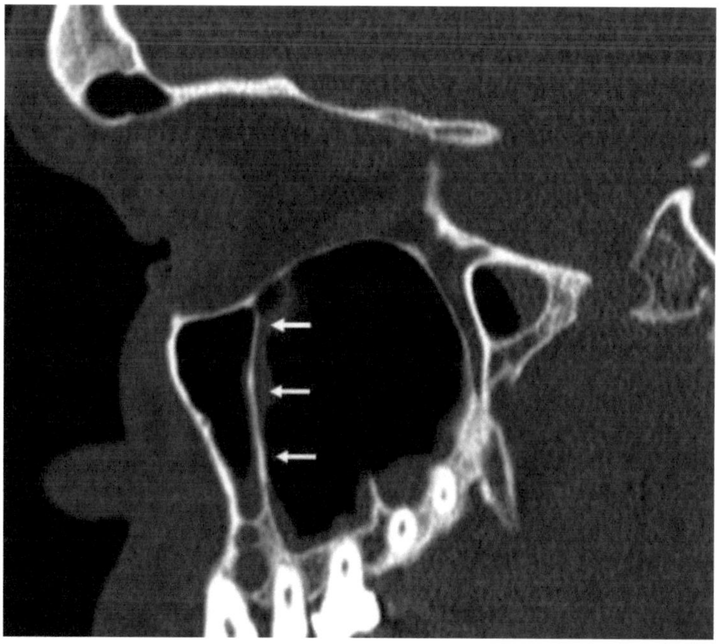

Figure 11. Parasagittal CT scan at the level of left maxillary sinus, showing a bony maxillary sinus septum (arrows). Large sinus septum could compromise the drainage of the sinus.

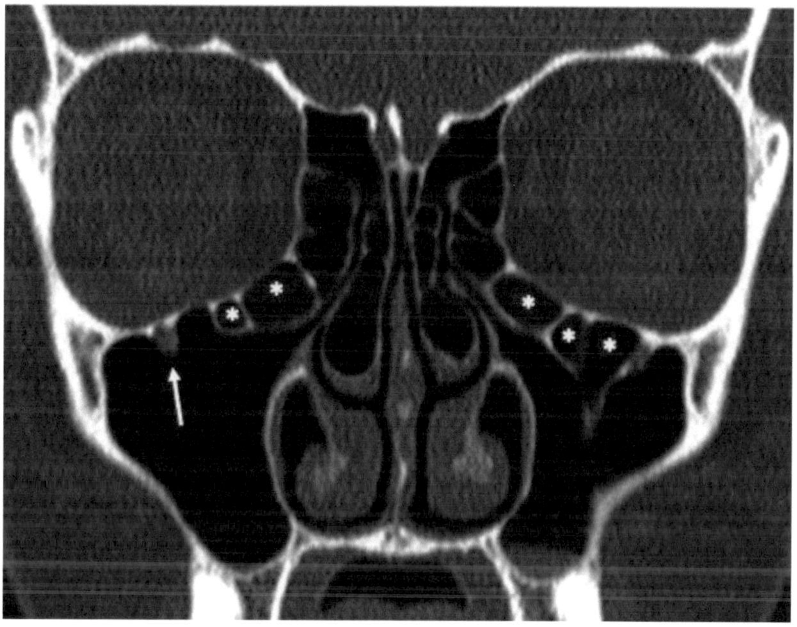

Figure 12. Coronal CT scan illustrates multiple bilateral infraorbital air cells "Haller cells" (asterisks). Any extension of ethmoid pneumatization at the orbital floor and lateral to lamina papyracea is labeled as Haller cell. Note how these cells significantly narrow the maxillary ostia bilaterally. Also, the infraorbital nerve canal on the right side is in the normal position; however, there is a complete dehiscence of its inferior bony wall (arrow). Patient is having large bilateral concha bullosa as well, which can further affect the ostiomeatal unit patency.

4.5. Blood supply, innervation, and lymphatic drainage

Maxillary sinus receives its blood supply by small arteries from the sphenopalatine, infraorbital, greater palatine, facial, pterygopalatine, posterior lateral nasal, and posterior superior alveolar arteries. Veins accompany these vessels drain to the facial vein and to the pterygoid plexus.

The innervations are from the maxillary division (V2) of trigeminal nerve through various branches, namely superior alveolar (posterior, middle, and anterior), greater palatine, and infraorbital nerves. While the area of the ostium is the most sensitive portion, the main part of the sinus is being relatively insensitive.

The lymphatic drainage is through the infraorbital foramen or the ostium to the submandibular node.

5. Ethmoid sinus

The ethmoid bone consists of five components: crista galli, cribriform plate, perpendicular plate, and two ethmoidal labyrinths. Each ethmoid labyrinth projects laterally from the side of the perpendicular plate. Each ethmoidal labyrinth consists of middle and superior turbinates, ethmoid air cells, and a thin paper-like lateral surface called "the lamina papyracea." The lamina papyracea forms a large part of the medial orbital wall as well.

The ethmoid air cells are divided by the basal lamella of middle turbinate into anterior and posterior ethmoid sinuses. The ethmoidal labyrinth does not have its own roof, and the roof of the sinus is formed by the orbital plate of frontal bone "Fovea ethmoidalis" [25].

Unlike the other sinuses, ethmoid sinus is not formed by a single air cell, instead it is divided by bony septa into variable number of air cells. Anterior ethmoid contains more air cells than the posterior ethmoid; however, the posterior ethmoid air cells are larger. In adult individual, the average number is 3–7 air cells in the anterior ethmoid sinus, and 2–4 in the posterior ethmoid. Each air cell drains through its own ostium, with anterior ethmoid air cells drain into the middle meatus and the posterior ones drain into the superior meatus [26].

5.1. Ethmoid bulla

The ethmoid bulla is the largest air cell of anterior ethmoid sinus. It extends from the lamina papyracea laterally and bulges medially into the middle meatus. The ostium of the ethmoid bulla often located on the upper margin of the posterior wall and drains into the middle meatus. Ethmoid bulla can be of variable sizes; however, occasionally "about 8% of the population," it might be underdeveloped [27].

A rare anatomical variation of the ethmoid bulla, when it is non-pneumatized. In this case, there will be a bony projection from the lamina papyracea known as "torus lateralis." Surgeon must be aware of this anatomical variant during endoscopic sinus surgery to prevent any unintentional orbital penetration [28].

5.2. Anterior ethmoidal artery

The anterior ethmoidal artery is one of the critical structures within the ethmoid sinus. After branching from the ophthalmic artery within the orbit, it pierces the upper portion of the lamina, then crosses the roof of anterior ethmoid sinus within a bony canal (approximately 2–3 mm behind the face of the ethmoid bulla). After crossing the sinus, it pierces the lateral lamella to enter the olfactory fossa. Then descends into nasal cavity through a slit on the side of the crista galli (**Figure 13A**).

The anterior ethmoidal artery foramen in the lamina papyracea is located about 24 mm posterior to the anterior lacrimal crest. The ophthalmic artery gives off another branch "the posterior ethmoidal artery" as well, which enters the posterior ethmoidal foramen 36 mm posterior to the anterior lacrimal crest [29].

Occasionally, the anterior ethmoidal artery bony canal might be dehiscent or totally absent, and the artery is suspended on the mucosa of the sinus (**Figure 13B**). The importance of preoperative identification of this condition cannot be stressed enough to avoid injuring the artery during operating endoscopically on the ethmoid sinus.

5.3. Development of the ethmoid sinus

Formation of the ethmoid sinus starts in fetal life. At birth, the sinus is present and can be identified radiologically. There is a rapid pneumatization between the first year and the age

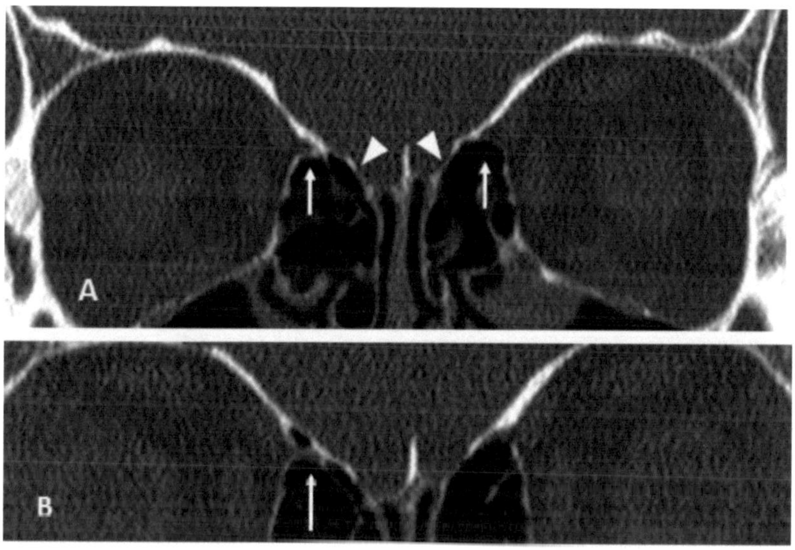

Figure 13. Coronal CT scan showing (A) the anterior ethmoidal artery canals while crossing the roof of ethmoid sinuses (arrows). The anterior ethmoidal artery foramen can be identified on the radiological imaging as a beak at the medial orbital wall. (B) Dehiscence of the bony canal and the anterior ethmoidal artery is suspended within the sinus on right side (arrow). Note the dehiscence of the inferior wall of the bony canal on the left side (arrowheads) indicate the thin lateral lamellae of the cribriform plate.

of four. Then it grows slowly till reaching the adult appearance by the age of 12. The clinical implication of the ethmoid sinus course of development is that the sinus could be the source of orbital infection in pediatric age group. And it is amenable to be surgically drained in this age group as well [30].

5.4. Anatomical variations of the ethmoid sinus

- **Agger nasi cell:** Makes the most anterior ethmoid air cells. Formed by an extension of the ethmoid air cell pneumatization into the lacrimal bone, and it is found as a prominence anterior to the vertical (anterior) attachment of middle turbinate (**Figure 14**). Their incidence is high, seen in about 93% of the population. Its size has a direct effect on the drainage of frontal sinus [31].

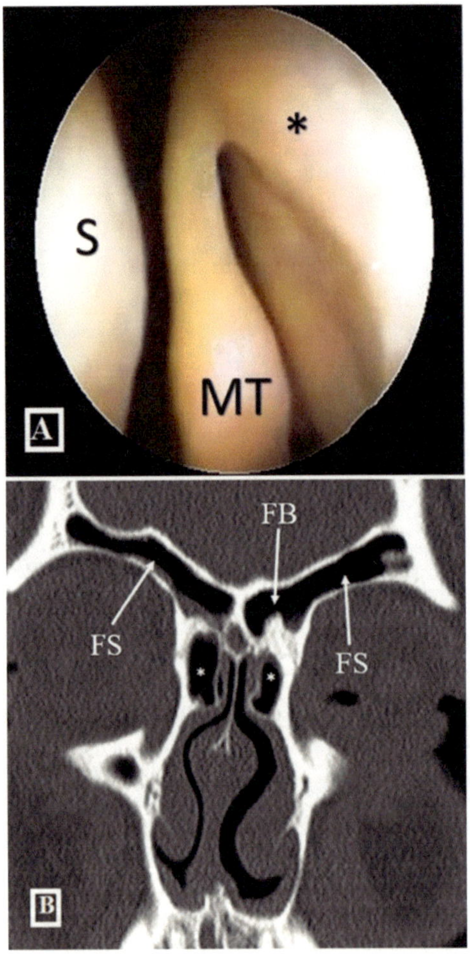

Figure 14. (A) Endoscopic picture showing the left agger nasi air cell as a prominence just anterior to the neck of the middle turbinate (asterisk). S, nasal septum; MT, middle turbinate. (B) Coronal CT scan at anterior level, showing bilateral agger nasi air cells (asterisk). Note the frontal sinuses (FS) and the frontal beak (FB) which corresponds to the frontal sinus ostium "refer to frontal sinus section".

- **Suprabullar recess and retrobullar recess:** When the upper border of the ethmoid bulla is not reaching the skull base, the space formed between them is referred to as "suprabullar recess." And when there is a space between the posterior wall of the bulla and the basal lamella, posteriorly, this space is called "retrobullar recess" (**Figure 15**).

- **Suprabullar cell:** An ethmoid air cell lies above the ethmoid bulla, so the superior border is related to the anterior cranial fossa. This cell is limited to the posterior portion of the frontal recess and does not extend to the frontal sinus (which differentiates it from the frontal bullar cell, the latter does extend to the frontal sinus). So, the anterior border of the suprabullar cell is made by the frontal recess (**Figure 5**).

- **Supraorbital cell:** A lateral extension of pneumatization from the suprabullar recess into the orbital plate of frontal bone over the orbit (**Figure 16**). Literature report 15% as an incidence of the supraorbital cell occurrence in the population.

  The anatomical significance of the supraorbital cell is that if it is large it can displace the anterior ethmoidal artery posteriorly. In addition, during endoscopic sinus surgery, it can be mistaken as the frontal sinus [32].

- Occasionally, small focal corticated defects in the lamina papyracea can be seen in up to 0.5–10% of the population; however, they are not clinically significant [33].

- **Sphenoethmoidal cell (Onodi's cell):** When the posterior ethmoid air cells pneumatized further posteriorly, and extend superiorly and laterally to sphenoid sinus, it is called the sphenoethmoidal cell or Onodi's cell. This can be explained by the fact that the ethmoid air cells are developed and pneumatized earlier than the sphenoid sinus, so they have a room

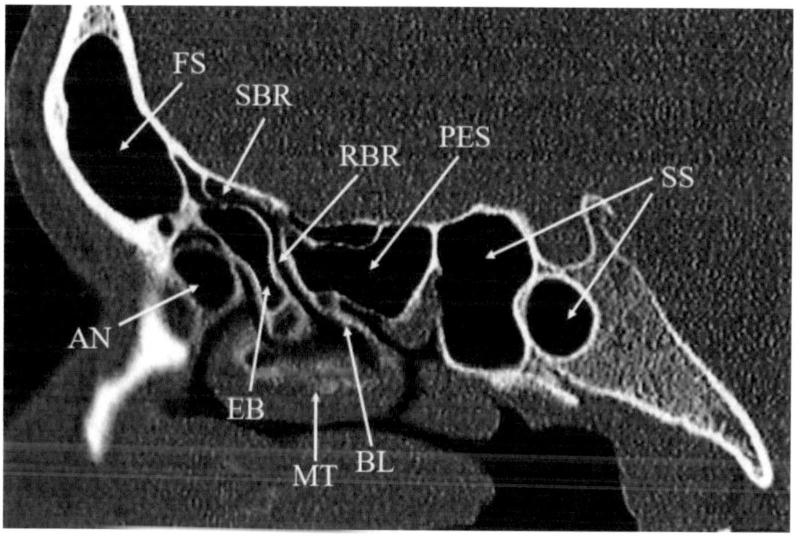

Figure 15. Parasagittal CT scan showing an ethmoid bulla (EB) that is not extending superiorly to the skull base, the gap created between it and the skull base is known as the suprabullar recess (SBR). Also, note that there is a gap between the posterior bullar wall and the basal lamella (BL), which is referred to as the retrobullar recess (RBR). FS, frontal sinus; AN, Agger nasi air cell; MT, middle turbinate; SS, right and left sphenoid sinuses. PES, posterior ethoid sinus.

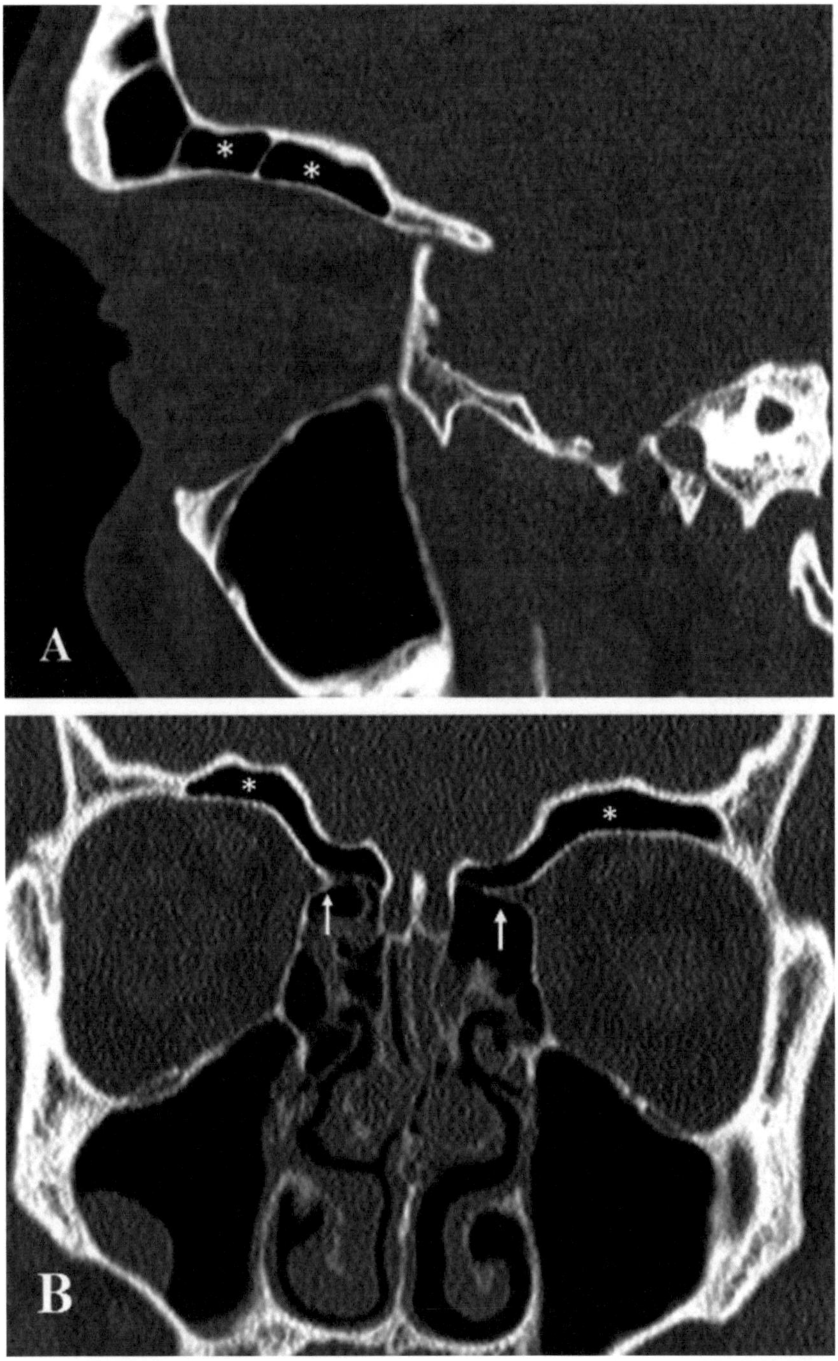

Figure 16. (A) Parasagittal CT scan showing an extension of pneumatization over the orbit (asterisks). (B) Coronal image of same study, showing bilateral supraorbital air cell (asterisks), note the anterior ethmoidal artery canal "arrows" is crossing between the anterior ethmoid sinus and the supraorbital air cell, which subjected the artery to a great risk during endoscopic sinus surgery while approaching these air cells.

to extend posteriorly. The incidence of the sphenoethmoidal cell ranges from 3.4 to 14% in the literature [34]. The significance of this air cell is that it is closely related to the optic nerve on its superolateral wall, and the nerve can even be engulfed within the air cell as well (**Figure 17**).

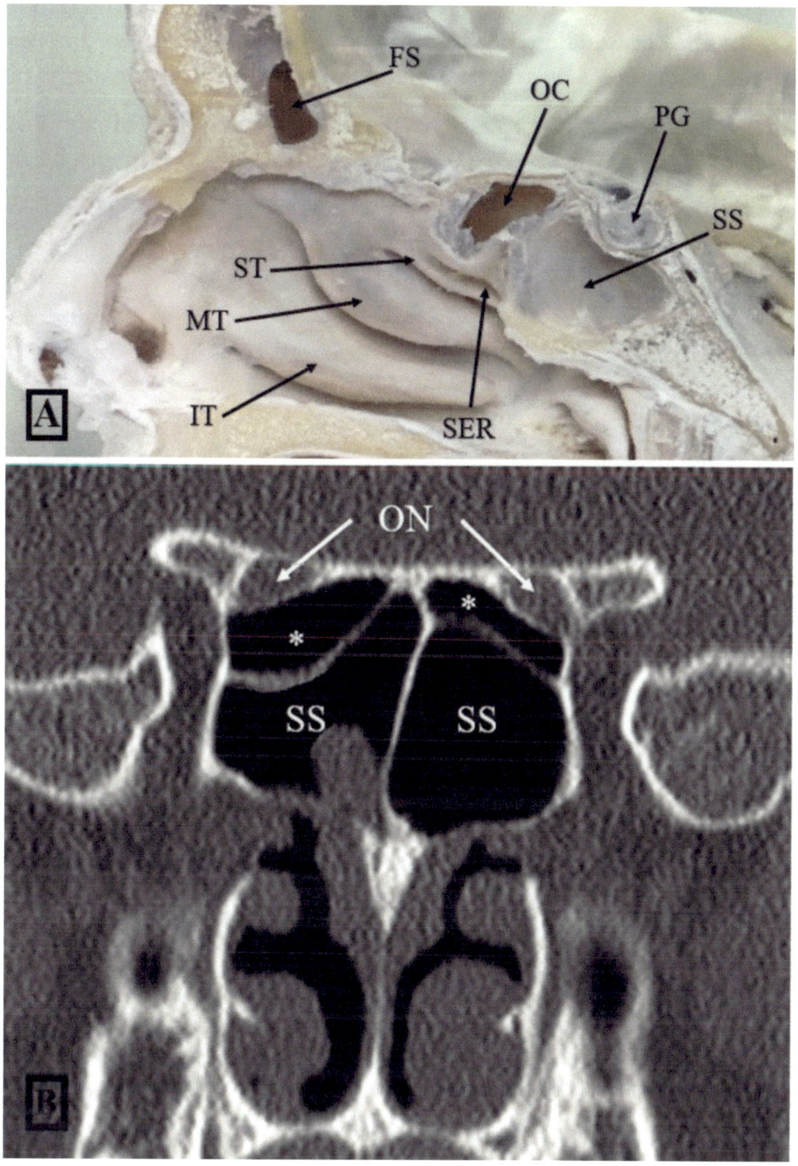

Figure 17. (A) Parasagittal gross picture showing how the Onodi's cell (OC) is extending posteriorly over the sphenoid sinus (SS). Note that Onodi's cell drains into the superior meatus, in contrary to the sphenoid sinus which drains into the sphenoethmoid recess (SER) lateral to the superior turbinate (ST). IT, inferior turbinate; MT, middle turbinate; FS, frontal sinus; PG, pituitary gland. (B) Coronal CT scan view at posterior level showing bilateral Onodi's cells (asterisks). Note how the optic nerve canals (ON) are closely related to the superolateral walls of the Onodi's cells. SS, sphenoid sinus.

- **Pneumatized crista galli:** Seen in 13% of individuals. The pneumatization extends from the frontal sinuses. Rarely can obstruct the frontal ostium [35].

5.5. Blood supply, innervation, and lymphatic drainage

Anterior and posterior ethmoid sinuses receive blood supply by branches from the supraorbital, anterior, and posterior ethmoidal and sphenopalatine arteries. The venous drainage is via the accompanying veins to the superior ophthalmic vein or pterygopalatine plexus.

The innervation is by anterior and posterior ethmoidal nerves of the ophthalmic division (V1) and the posterior nasal branch of the maxillary division (V2) of the trigeminal nerve.

The lymphatic drainage of the anterior ethmoid sinus is to the submandibular nodes, and the posterior ethmoid sinus drains to the retropharyngeal nodes.

6. Frontal sinus

There are two sinuses extending in the squamous part of the frontal bone. They are separated by bony septum because each sinus (right and left) develops independently; they are expected to be asymmetrically pneumatized. The larger sinus may pass across the midline and overlap the other.

Sinus's anterior and posterior walls are called outer and inner frontal table, respectively. The inner table is a relative thin bony plate that separates frontal sinus from the anterior cranial fossa posteriorly. On the other hand, the outer table is a considerable thick bony wall [36]. On the posterior wall (inner table) of the sinus, there are venous drainage channels called "foramina of Breschet." These foramina have clinical significance in their role in spreading the infection from the sinus toward intracranially. Also, these foramina act as sites of mucosal invagination within the bone, so failing to completely remove the mucosa in these sites during the sinus obliteration procedure may predispose to the development of mucocele. The floor of each frontal sinus forms the anterior roof of the orbit. The floor consisted of a thin bone which can be eroded by the mucocele.

6.1. Frontal ostium and frontal recess (frontal sinus drainage pathway)

Frontal sinus ostium is located at the posteromedial part of sinus's floor. The frontal sinus drainage pathway has an hour-glass shape, with the narrowest point of this pathway corresponds to "the frontal beak" which represents the frontal sinus ostium (**Figure 18**A). Therefore, what lies superior to the frontal beak is frontal sinus, and what lies inferior to the beak is frontal recess [37]. The thickness of the frontal beak (frontonasal process of the maxilla) will determine the size and patency the frontal sinus ostium.

Frontal recess is like an inverted funnel with its apex formed by the frontal sinus ostium. The frontal recess is not a structure by itself, rather it is formed by walls of the surrounding structures. Boundaries of frontal recess are as follows: from the anterior and inferior side, the posterior wall of agger nasi cell; from the posterior side, the face of ethmoid bulla;

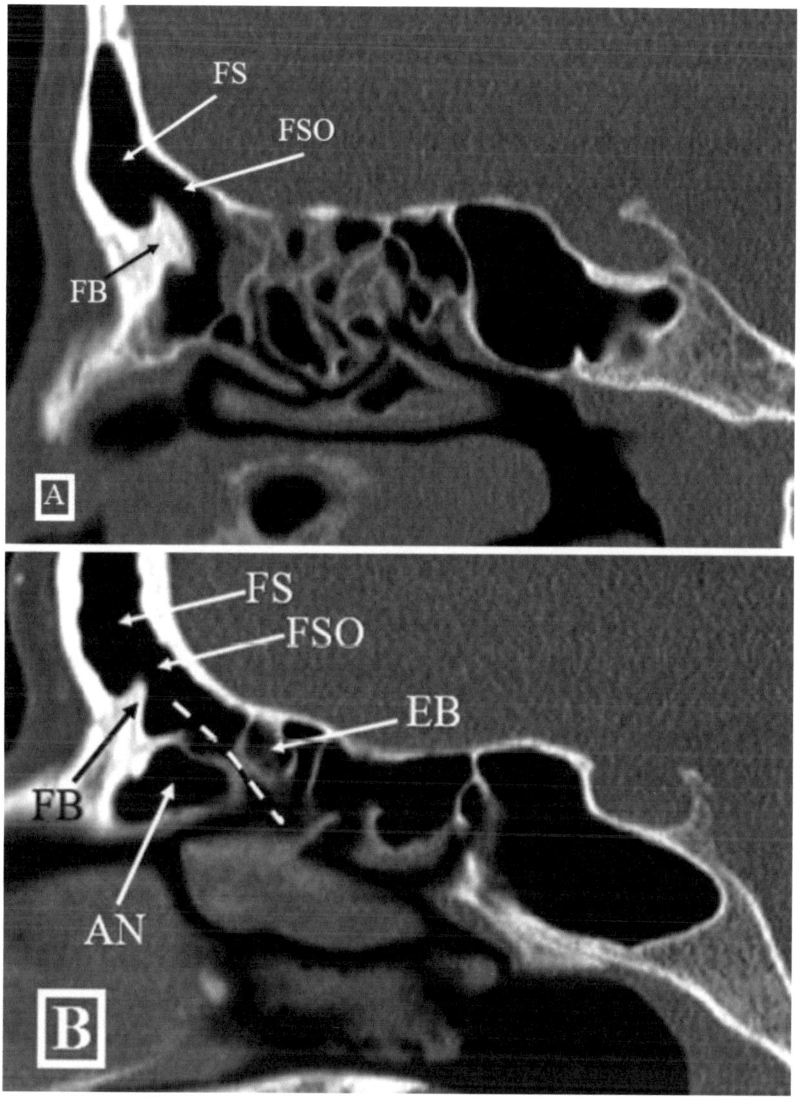

Figure 18. Parasagittal CT scan images. (A) Prominent frontal beak (FB) which corresponds to the level of the frontal sinus ostium (FSO). Superior to the beak is the frontal sinus (FS). (B) A relatively small frontal beak (FB), which is often associated with large agger nasi air cell (AN). Note that the large agger nasi cell causing a significant narrowing of the frontal recess (dashed line). As agger nasi cell forms the anterior wall of the recess, ethmoid bulla (EB) forms the posterior wall. So, any enlargement or pathology affecting either cells could compromise the patency of the frontal recess.

lateral boundary is formed by the lamina papyracea; medial side formed by the lateral wall of olfactory fossa and the upper portion of middle turbinate; and superiorly, comes the fovea ethmoidalis.

Depending on the superior attachment of the uncinate process, the frontal sinus drainage pathway drains into the middle meatus or the ethmoid infundibulum (as mentioned in the uncinate process section) [38].

6.2. The relationship between frontal beak and agger nasi cell size

When agger nasi cell is small, the frontal beak becomes prominent and narrows the ostium. In contrary, the large agger nasi cell results in a small frontal beak which means wider frontal sinus ostium. However, the large agger nasi cell might compromise the frontal sinus drainage pathway at the level of frontal recess, inferiorly (**Figure 18B**) [39].

6.3. Anatomical variations of frontal sinus

- Frontal sinus aplasia (totally absent) is found in 5% of the population (**Figure 19**). And hypoplastic frontal sinus is found in 4%.
- **Frontoethmoidal cells (Frontal cells):** Classification of frontal cells was first described by Kuhn [40]. However, later Wormald modified the frontal cells classification [41]. (This chapter reviews the modified classification by Wormald.) They were classified into four groups as follows:

    Type 1 frontal cell: Single frontal recess cell (above agger nasi cell and below the frontal ostium) (**Figure 20A**).

    Type 2 frontal cells: Two or more cells in frontal recess (above agger nasi cell and below the frontal ostium) (**Figure 20B**).

    Type 3 frontal cell: Single cell above the agger nasi with extension into the frontal sinus through the frontal ostium but not exceeding 50% of the vertical height of the ipsilateral frontal sinus (**Figure 20C**).

    Type 4 frontal cell: Either single cell above the agger nasi with extension into the frontal sinus through the frontal ostium, and exceeding 50% of the vertical height of the ipsilateral frontal sinus, or an isolated cell within the frontal sinus (above the frontal ostium) (**Figure 20D**).

- **Frontal bullar cell**: Single cell extends from the suprabullar region along the posterior wall of frontal recess and extends into the frontal sinus, superiorly. This differentiates it from

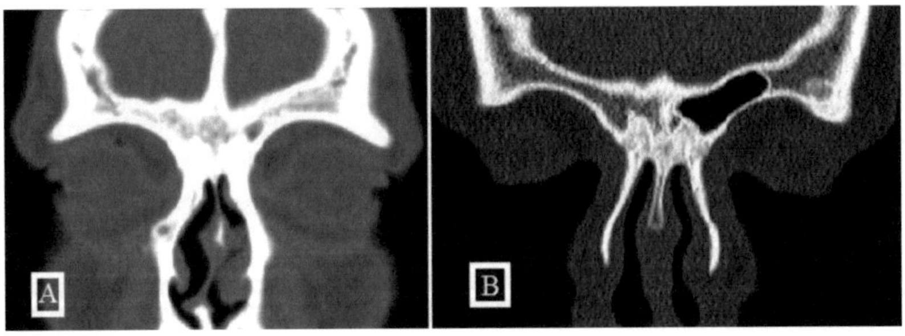

Figure 19. Coronal CT scan. (A) Bilateral aplastic frontal sinuses. (B) Because each frontal sinus develops independently, a variant like unilateral aplastic frontal sinus can occur.

http://dx.doi.org/10.5772/intechopen.69089

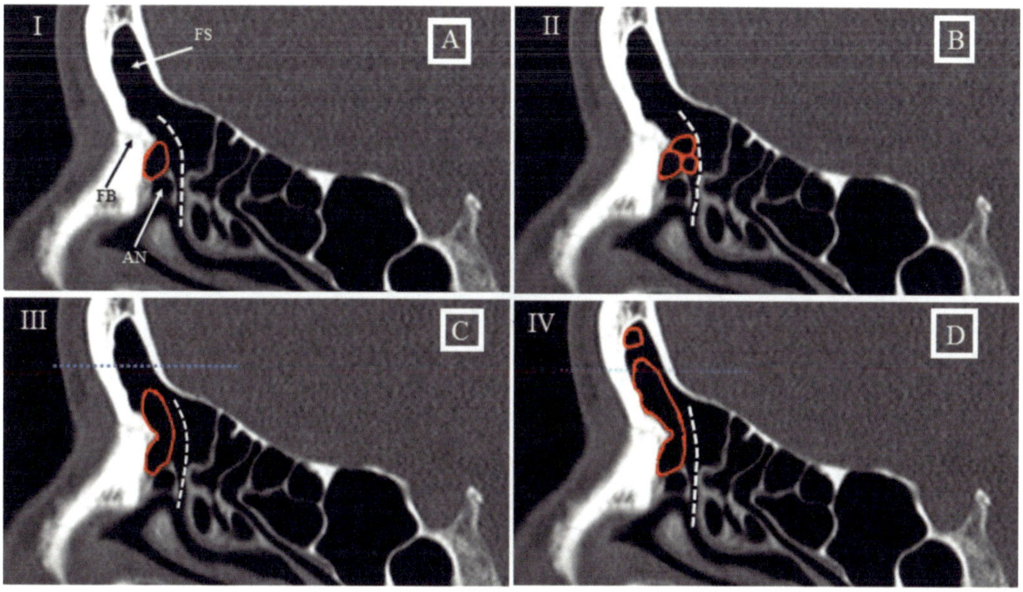

Figure 20. Parasagittal diagram demonstrating four types of the frontoethmoidal "frontal" cells (red). FS, frontal sinus; FB, frontal beak "corresponding to the frontal ostium"; AN, agger nasi cell; blue dashed line represents the midway of the frontal sinus vertical length.

the suprabullar cell, which does not extend into the frontal sinus. The posterior wall of the frontal bullar cell is related to anterior cranial fossa, and its anterior wall is related to frontal sinus (**Figure 21**). Caution must be taken during opening this cell not to cause unintentional trauma to anterior skull base.

- **Frontal intersinus septal cell:** Occasionally, the intersinus septum is pneumatized forming an intersinus air cell, which might be communicating with either one of the frontal sinuses or could be completely an isolated air cell. It might compromise the frontal sinus ostium patency [42] (**Figure 22**).

6.4. Air cells that might affect the patency of the frontal ostium or the recess

(1) Agger nasi cell; (2) Ethmoid bulla; (3) Suprabullar cell; (4) Frontal bullar cell; (5) Frontoethmoidal cells (Frontal cells); (6) Frontal intersinus septal cell (**Figure 23**).

6.5. Development of frontal sinus

Frontal sinuses are the only sinuses that are not present at birth. They start pneumatization by the age of two and reach the orbital roof by the age of 5–7. By age of 12, they reach the adult size [3]. The clinical application of the frontal sinus development process is that external trephination procedure is contraindicated before the developing sinus reaches the level of orbital roof because of the risk of intracranial penetration.

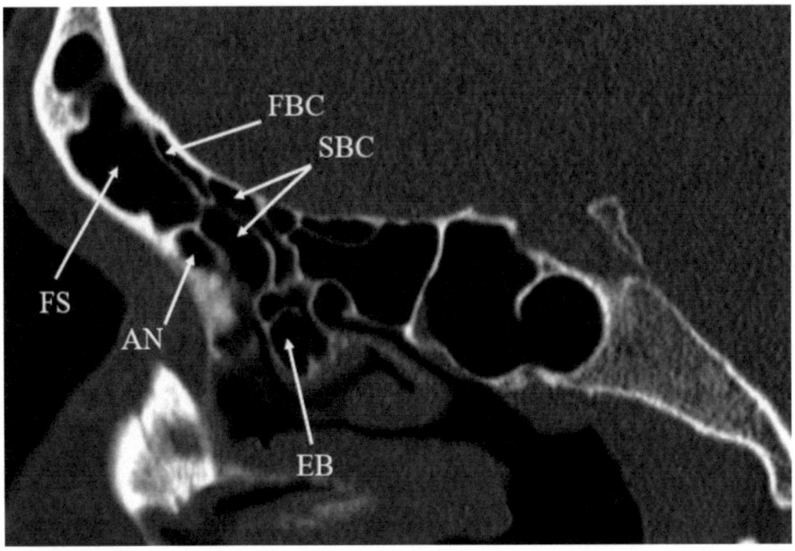

Figure 21. Parasagittal CT scan showing frontal bullar cell (FBC). Note that the posterior border of the cell is related to the anterior cranial fossa. And the frontal sinus (FS) is making the anterior border. The suprabullar cells (SBC) are limited to the frontal recess and are not extending to frontal sinus. AN, Agger nasi; EB, ethmoid bulla.

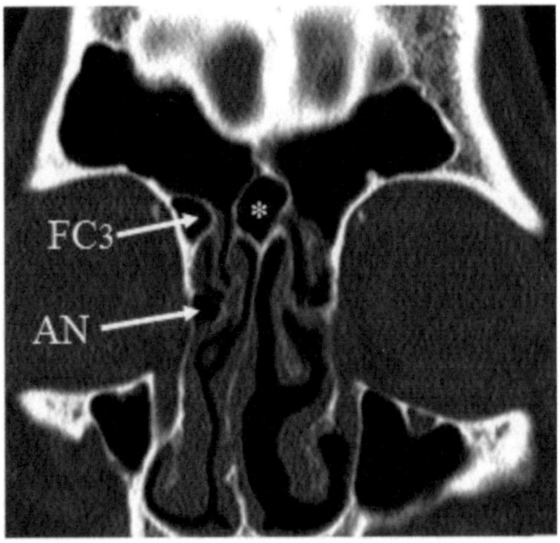

Figure 22. Coronal CT scan showing frontal intersinus septal air cell (asterisk). Note the frontal cell type 3 on the right frontal sinus (FC3). Frontal sinus ostium might be compromised because of the impact of either of these two cells. AN, Agger nasi cell.

6.6. Blood supply, innervation, and lymphatic drainage

Frontal sinus receives blood supply from the supratrochlear and supraorbital arteries (branching from ophthalmic artery). Venous drainage is by the superior ophthalmic and diploic veins. Lymph drainage is across the face to the submandibular nodes. Frontal sinus receives innervation from the supratrochlear and supraorbital nerves.

http://dx.doi.org/10.5772/intechopen.69089

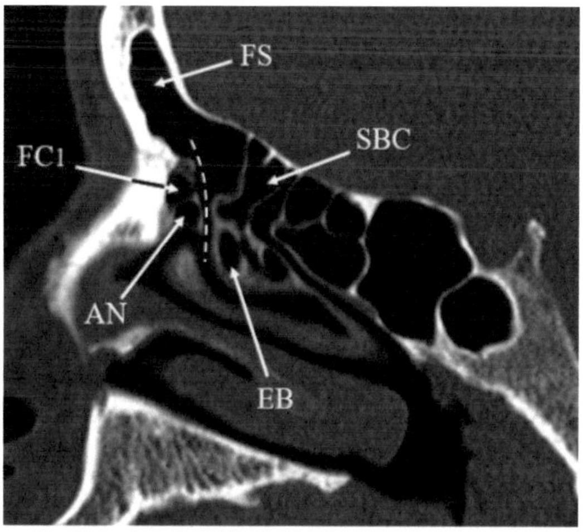

Figure 23. Parasagittal CT view of the frontal recess (dashed line). Note that anterior to the frontal recess are the agger nasi cell (AN) and frontoethmoidal cell "frontal cell" type 1 (FC1). And posterior to the recess are the ethmoid bulla (EB) and the suprabullar cell (SBC). Expanding of any of these air cells could have an impact on the patency of the frontal recess. Also, other air cells like frontal bullar cell or frontal intersinus septal cell could compromise frontal sinus drainage pathway at the ostium level.

7. Sphenoid sinus

Sphenoid sinuses occupy the body of sphenoid bone. Classically, there are two asymmetrical sinuses separated by off-midline intersphenoid bony septum.

7.1. Sphenoid sinus ostium and posterior septal artery

Sphenoid sinus drains into the sphenoethmoidal recess through a single sphenoid ostium in the sinus's anterior wall, which opens medial to superior turbinate. Typically, the ostium is located in the medial portion of sphenoidal face, about 10–12 mm superior to the upper border of the choana. Also, it can be located be measuring 7 cm from anterior nasal spine at an angle of 30° with the nasal floor. The posteroinferior end (the tail) of superior turbinate can be used to locate the ostium, which typically would be just superomedial to the tail of superior turbinate [43].

Inferior to sphenoid natural ostium, the posterior septal artery (a branch of sphenopalatine artery) crosses the sphenoid face from the lateral nasal wall to the posterior end of nasal septum. Either it bifurcates into superior and inferior branches before crossing (65%) or crosses as main artery then bifurcates (35%). Even if it bifurcates before crossing, both branches pass inferior to the ostium. The average distance between the sphenoid ostium and the posterior septal artery or its superior branch is about 5 mm. Because of that, during widening the ostium, it is safer to dissect and widen the sphenoid ostium horizontally and superiorly. Alternatively, to use the electrocautery if the ostium will be widening more than 5 mm inferiorly [44].

7.2. Vital structures surrounding the sphenoid sinus

Vital structures such as pituitary gland, optic nerves, cavernous sinuses and carotid arteries, maxillary divisions (V2) of the trigeminal nerves within the foramina rotundum, and vidian canals are closely related to the sphenoid body. Depending on the degree of pneumatization of the sinus, these structures could be seen as indentations on the sinus's roof and walls, internally.

Roof of the sinus is related to the pituitary gland and middle cranial fossa. Posteriorly lie the pons and the posterior cranial fossa. The optic nerve canal crosses the corner formed by the roof and the lateral wall on the posterior portion of the sinus on each side. On the posterolateral walls, internal carotid artery canals (cavernous segment) will be seen as bony prominences. Within the lateral sphenoid walls, the maxillary division of trigeminal nerves pass through the foramina rotundum toward the pterygopalatine fossae in both sides. Vidian nerves cross the lateral sides of the sinus floor within the vidian canals "pterygoid canals" (**Figure 24**).

7.3. Anatomical variations of sphenoid sinus

- **Sphenoid sinus pneumatization:** Depending on the degree of pneumatization, sphenoid sinus is classified into three types [45].
    - **Conchal type:** The degree of pneumatization is limited to the anterior portion of the sphenoid body and not reaching the level of the anterior wall of sella turcica. Seen in 1–4% of individuals (**Figure 25A**).
    - **Presellar type:** Pneumatization extends up to the vertical level of the anterior wall of sella turcica but not beyond that. Found in 35–40% of the population (**Figure 25B**).

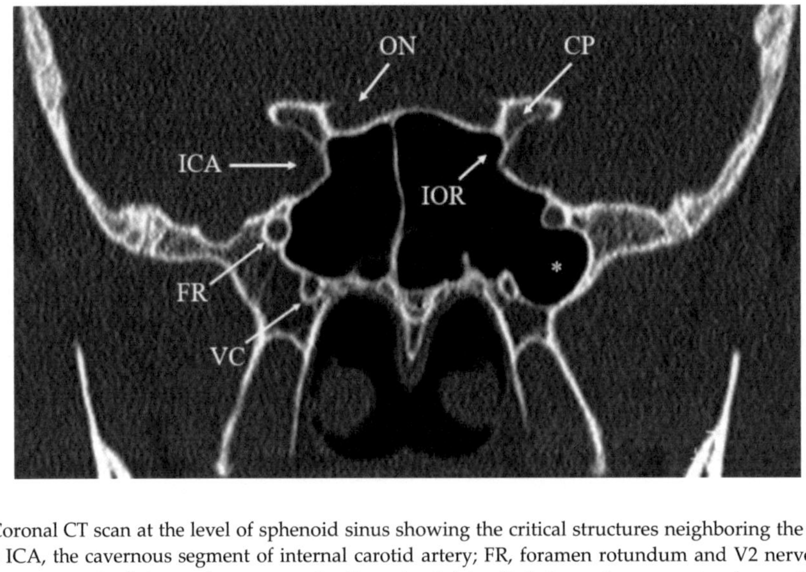

Figure 24. Coronal CT scan at the level of sphenoid sinus showing the critical structures neighboring the sinuses. ON, optic nerve; ICA, the cavernous segment of internal carotid artery; FR, foramen rotundum and V2 nerve; VC, vidian canal. In hyperpneumatized sinus, when pneumatization extends laterally between foramen rotundum and vidian canal, creating a recess known as the lateral recess (asterisk). When pneumatization extends below the optic canal "between optic canal and internal carotid artery" resulted in infraoptic "opticocarotid" recess (IOR). CP, anterior clinoid process.

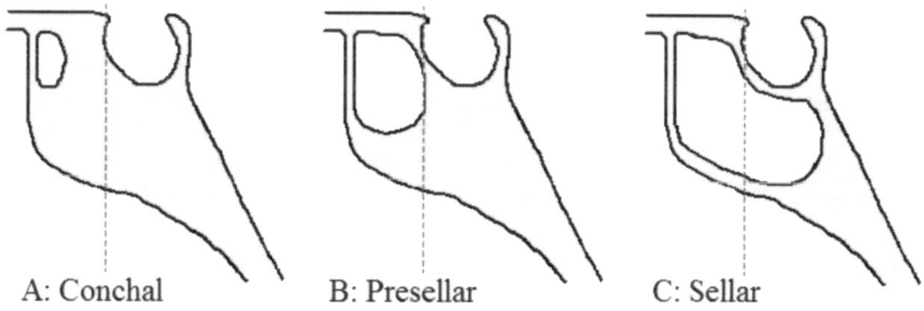

Figure 25. Sagittal view showing the types and degree of sphenoid sinus pneumatization related to the anterior wall of sella turcica (dashed line). (A) Conchal, when not reaching the vertical level of the anterior wall of sella turcica. (B) Presellar, when reaches but not beyond it. (C) Sellar, pneumatization beyond the anterior wall of sella turcica. Note the presence of a good density of cortical bone anterior to the pituitary fossa in conchal type, making procedures like endoscopic trans-sphenoid hypophysectomy, relatively contraindicated.

- **Sellar type:** Pneumatization extends beyond the level of the anterior wall of sella turcica below the pituitary fossa (**Figure 25C**) and might reach posterior to the sella turcica "occasionally called postsellar type" [46]. The sellar type is the most common one, seen in 55–60% of the population.

  Sphenoid sinus agenesis: When non-pneumatized sinus, it is found in less than 0.7% of the population.

  Sphenoid sinus agenesis or the conchal type are relative contraindications for endoscopic trans-sphenoid skull base approach.

- **Optic nerve canal dehiscence:** In 4% of cases, the bony canal is having a focal dehiscence and only sinus mucosa with neural sheath are separating the nerve from the sinus. In 78% of cases, the thickness of the wall of optic canal that separates it from the sinus is less than 0.5 mm [47] (**Figure 26B**).
- **Internal carotid artery canal dehiscence:** When areas of the medial side of bony canal separating the sinus from the artery are defected, putting the internal carotid artery at risk during the endoscopic sphenoid surgery. It was reported in literature a rate between 8 and 25% as the incidence of this variant [47, 48].

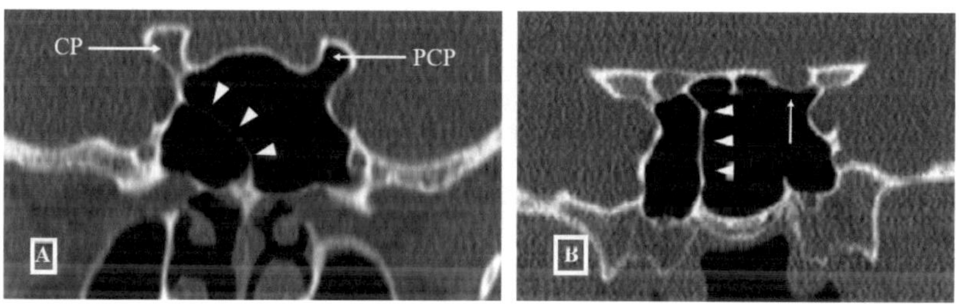

Figure 26. Coronal CT scan of the sphenoid sinus showing (A) Deviated sphenoid intersinus septum and attached to the right internal carotid artery canal (arrowheads). Also, note the extension of pneumatization to the left anterior clinoid process (PCP: Pneumatized clinoid process). Right normal anterior clinoid process (CP) indicated for comparison. (B) Deviated intersphenoid septum which attached to right optic canal (arrowheads). Note how thin can be the inferior bony wall of optic nerve canal, on the left side (arrow).

- The sphenoid intersinus septum occasionally deviates off the midline and has an insertion on the internal carotid artery bony canal or the optic canal. Excessive traction on the septum should be avoided, in these cases, not to cause avulsion of the bony wall (**Figure 26**).
- **Pneumatized posterior nasal septum:** Might be from an extension of air from the sphenoid sinus or crista galli. Rarely this cause narrowing of the sphenoethmoidal recess (**Figure 27**).
- **Supraoptic recess and infraoptic recess:** In hyperpneumatized sphenoid sinus, when pneumatization reaches superiorly and inferiorly to the optic canal, it will result in these two recesses, respectively. Because the infraoptic recess lies between the optic canal and internal carotid artery canal, also known as "opticocarotid recess" (**Figure 24**). In addition, pneumatization can extend from the infraoptic recess to the anterior clinoid process (**Figure 26A**).
- **Lateral recess:** When pneumatization extensively extends inferolaterally between the maxillary (V2) and vidian nerves, it creates this recess (**Figure 24**).

7.4. Development of the sphenoid sinus

At birth, it is not more than a small mucosal sac. Pneumatization starts around the third year of life. It gradually progresses until it reaches the adult size around the age of 14.

7.5. Blood supply, innervation, and lymphatic drainage

Arterial supply is from the posterior ethmoidal artery and posterior septal artery. Veins drain via the posterior ethmoidal vein to the superior ophthalmic vein. The sinus mucosa receives

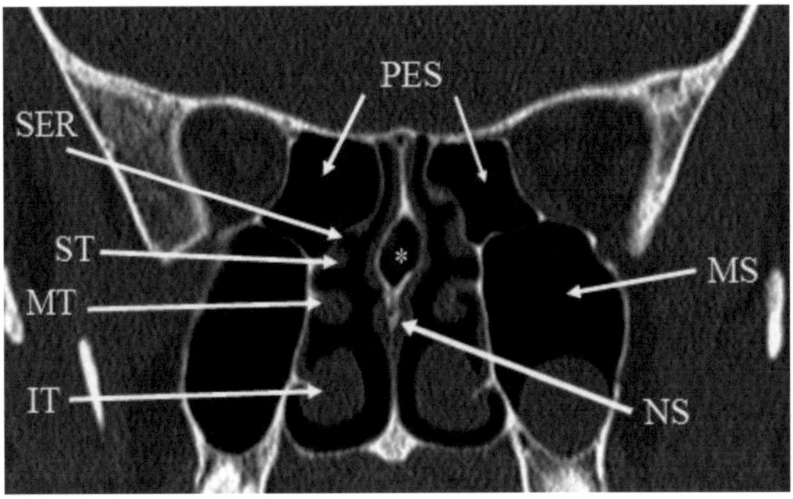

Figure 27. Coronal CT scan showing a pneumatized posterior nasal septum (asterisk). Note the proximity of sphenoethmoid recess (SER) to the pneumatized portion, which can be affected in extensive pneumatization. ST, tail of superior turbinate; NS, nasal septum; PES, posterior ethmoid sinus; MS, maxillary sinus; IT, inferior turbinate; MT, middle turbinate.

innervation from the posterior ethmoidal nerve and the orbital branch of pterygopalatine ganglion. The Lymph drains to the retropharyngeal nodes.

Author details

Abdulmalik S. Alsaied

Address all correspondence to: a.s.alsaied@gmail.com

Department of Otolaryngology, King Fahd Hospital of the University, University of Dammam, Dammam, Saudi Arabia

References

[1] Mygind N, Dahl R. Anatomy, physiology and function of the nasal cavities in health and disease. Advanced Drug Delivery Reviews. 1998;**29**(1):3-12

[2] Ogle OE, Weinstock RJ, Friedman E. Surgical anatomy of the nasal cavity and paranasal sinuses. Oral and Maxillofacial Surgery Clinics of North America. 2012;**24**(2):155-166

[3] Vaid S, Vaid N. Normal anatomy and anatomic variants of the paranasal sinuses on computed tomography. Neuroimaging Clinics of North America. 2015;**25**(4):527-548

[4] Sarna A, et al. Coronal imaging of the osteomeatal unit: Anatomy of 24 variants. Journal of Computer Assisted Tomography. 2002;**26**(1):153-157

[5] Zinreich SJ, et al. Concha bullosa: CT evaluation. Journal of Computer Assisted Tomography. 1988;**12**(5):778-784

[6] Beale TJ, Madani G, Morley SJ. Imaging of the paranasal sinuses and nasal cavity: Normal anatomy and clinically relevant anatomical variants. Seminars in Ultrasound, CT and MRI. 2009;**30**(1):2-16

[7] Dogru H, et al. Pneumatized inferior turbinate. American Journal of Otolaryngology. 1999;**20**(2):139-141

[8] Khanobthamchai K, et al. The secondary middle turbinate. Journal of Otolaryngology. 1991;**20**(6):412-413

[9] Akoungur EH, et al. CT demonstration of accessory nasal turbinates: Secondary middle turbinate and bifid inferior turbinate. European Journal of Radiology. 1999;**31**(3):174-176

[10] Vaid S, et al. An imaging checklist for pre-FESS CT: Framing a surgically relevant report. Clinical Radiology. 2011;**66**(5):459-470

[11] Kennedy DW, Zinreich SJ. The functional endoscopic approach to inflammatory sinus disease: current perspectives and technique modifications. American Journal of Rhinology. 1988;**2**(3):89-96

[12] Bolger WE, Parsons DS, Butzin CA. Paranasal sinus bony anatomic variations and mucosal abnormalities: CT analysis for endoscopic sinus surgery. The Laryngoscope. 1991; **101**(1):56-64

[13] Keros P. On the practical value of differences in the level of the lamina cribrosa of the ethmoid. Zeitschrift fur Laryngologie, Rhinologie, Otologie und ihre Grenzgebiete. 1962;**41**:809-813

[14] Lund VJ, et al. European position paper on the anatomical terminology of the internal nose and paranasal sinuses. Rhinology. 2014;**Suppl 24**:1-34

[15] Lee HY, et al. Surgical anatomy of the sphenopalatine artery in lateral nasal wall. The Laryngoscope. 2002;**112**(10):1813-1818

[16] Yoon JH, et al. Fontanelle and uncinate process in the lateral wall of the human nasal cavity. The Laryngoscope. 2000;**110**(2):281

[17] Gosau M, et al. Maxillary sinus anatomy: A cadaveric study with clinical implications. The Anatomical Record. 2009;**292**(3):352-354

[18] Bergh J, et al. Anatomical aspects of sinus floor elevations. Clinical Oral Implants Research. 2000;**11**(3):256-265

[19] Whittet HB. Infraorbital nerve dehiscence: the anatomic cause of maxillary sinus "vacuum headache"? Otolaryngology—Head and Neck Surgery. 1992;**107**(1):21-28

[20] Kubal WS. Sinonasal anatomy. Neuroimaging Clinics of North America. 1998;**8**(1):143

[21] Lawson W, Patel ZM, Lin FY. The development and pathologic processes that influence maxillary sinus pneumatization. The Anatomical Record. 2008;**291**(11):1554-1563

[22] Jog M, McGarry GW. How frequent are accessory sinus ostia? The Journal of Laryngology and Otology. 2003;**117**(4):270-272

[23] Maestre-Ferrin L, et al. Maxillary sinus septa: A systematic review. Medicina Oral, Patología Oral y Cirugía Bucal. 2010;**15**(2):383-386

[24] Kantarci M, et al. Remarkable anatomic variations in paranasal sinus region and their clinical importance. European Journal of Radiology. 2004;**50**(3):296-302

[25] Stammberger H, Kennedy DW, Bolger W. Paranasal sinuses: Anatomic terminology and nomenclature. Annals of Otology, Rhinology and Laryngology. 1995;**167**:17-21

[26] Sargi ZB, Casiano RR. Surgical anatomy of the paranasal sinuses. In: Rhinologic and sleep apnea surgical techniques. Heidelberg: Springer Berlin; 2007. pp. 17-26

[27] Marquez S, et al. Development of the ethmoid sinus and extramural migration: The anatomical basis of this paranasal sinus. The Anatomical Record. 2008;**291**(11):1535-1553

[28] Polavaram R, et al. Anatomic variants and pearls–functional endoscopic sinus surgery. Otolaryngologic Clinics of North America. 2004;**37**(2):221-242

[29] Moon HJ, et al. Surgical anatomy of the anterior ethmoidal canal in ethmoid roof. The Laryngoscope. 2001;**111**(5):900-904

[30] Ballenger JJ, Snow Jr. JB. Anatomy and physiology of the nose and paranasal sinuses. Ballenger's Otorhinolaryngology Head and Neck Surgery. 2003;**16**:547-560

[31] Peter JW. The agger nasi cell: The key to understanding the anatomy of the frontal recess. Otolaryngology--Head and Neck Surgery. 2003;**129**(5):497-507

[32] Owen JR, Glen R, Kuhn FA. Supraorbital ethmoid cell. Otolaryngology--Head and Neck Surgery. 1997;**116**(2):254-261

[33] Moulin G, et al. Dehiscence of the lamina papyracea of the ethmoid bone: CT findings. American Journal of Neuroradiology. 1994;**15**(1):151-153

[34] Weinberger DG, et al. Surgical anatomy and variations of the Onodi cell. American Journal of Rhinology. 1996;**10**(6):365-370

[35] Som PM, et al. Crista galli pneumatization is an extension of the adjacent frontal sinuses. American Journal of Neuroradiology. 2009;**30**(1):31-33

[36] Duque CS, Casiano RR. Surgical anatomy and embryology of the frontal sinus. In: The Frontal Sinus. Heidelberg: Springer Berlin; 2005. pp. 21-31

[37] Kew J, et al. Multiplanar reconstructed computed tomography images improves depiction and understanding of the anatomy of the frontal sinus and recess. American Journal of Rhinology. 2002;**16**(2):119-123

[38] Lee D, Brody R, Har-El G. Frontal sinus outflow anatomy. American Journal of Rhinology. 1997;**11**(4):283-285

[39] Jacobs JB, et al. Role of the agger nasi cell in chronic frontal sinusitis. Annals of Otology, Rhinology and Laryngology. 1996;**105**(9):694-700

[40] Bent JP, Cuilty-Siller C, Kuhn FA. The frontal cell as a cause of frontal sinus obstruction. American Journal of Rhinology. 1994;**8**(4):185-191

[41] Wormald PJ. Surgery of the frontal recess and frontal sinus. Rhinology. 2005;**43**(2):82-85

[42] Som PM, Lawson W. The frontal intersinus septal air cell: A new hypothesis of its origin. American Journal of Neuroradiology. 2008;**29**(6):1215-1217

[43] Kim HU, et al. Surgical anatomy of the natural ostium of the sphenoid sinus. The Laryngoscope. 2001;**111**(9):1599-1602

[44] Zhang X, et al. Anatomy of the posterior septal artery with surgical implications on the vascularized pedicled nasoseptal flap. Head and Neck. 2015;**37**(10):1470-1476

[45] Sethi DS, Stanley RE, Pillay PK. Endoscopic anatomy of the sphenoid sinus and sella turcica. The Journal of Laryngology and Otology. 1995;**109**(10):951-955

[46] Guldner C, et al. Analysis of pneumatization and neurovascular structures of the sphenoid sinus using cone-beam tomography (CBT). Acta Radiologica. 2012;**53**(2):214-219

[47] Fujii K, Chambers SM, Rhoton Jr. AL. Neurovascular relationships of the sphenoid sinus: a microsurgical study. Journal of Neurosurgery. 1979;**50**(1):31-39

[48] Stammberger H, Lund V. Anatomy of the nose and paranasal sinuses. In: Gleeson M, Browning GG, Burton MJ, et al., editors. Scott-Brown's Otorhinolaryngology, head and neck surgery. Vol. 3. 7th ed. London: HodderArnold; 2008. pp. 1315-1343

Section 2

Dental Related Disease

Chapter 2

Maxillary Sinus Augmentation for Dental Implants

Gökhan Göçmen and Yasar Özkan

Additional information is available at the end of the chapter

http://dx.doi.org/10.5772/intechopen.69063

Abstract

Pneumatization of the maxillary sinus secondary to posterior maxillary tooth loss is an extremely common finding. Significant atrophy of the maxilla prevents dental implant placement in this region. Grafting the floor of the maxillary sinus has emerged as the most common surgical modality for correcting this inadequacy. Graft material is introduced into the space created inferior to the sinus membrane. Various grafting materials and techniques might be used in this procedure. The aim of this article is to review the essentials of maxillary sinus augmentation, clarify this procedure for otolaryngologists, explain its function, and describe the augmentation materials, techniques, and complications.

Keywords: maxillary, sinus, augmentation, dental, implant

1. Introduction

Paranasal sinuses are important anatomical structures in both medicine and dentistry. The maxillary sinus is the most relevant to dental practitioners due to its proximity to the posterior maxillary teeth. Dentists are often required to make a diagnosis concerning orofacial pain that may be sinogenic in origin. Maxillary sinus diseases can be observed coincidentally on radiographs from routine dental examinations and considered in differential diagnosis. Therefore, most dentists unintentionally take a look at the maxillary sinus of their patients.

The maxillary sinus or antrum of Highmore is generally avoided during dental surgeries. Communication or the development of space, between the maxillary sinus and the buccal cavity (oroantral) or between the nasal and buccal cavities (oronasal), has always been considered an undesired issue but is accepted as a complication when encountered after tooth extraction or any other oral-surgical procedure [1]. Disintegration or perforation of the sinus membrane is an unwelcome incident because of the need for additional surgeries.

In the instance of chronic oroantral fistula occurrence, the established fistula enables the passage between the oral cavity and the maxillary sinus. Consequently, the microbial flora can exchange and inflammation may occur with various possible consequences. This simple complication might lead to major problems, be handled easily, or recover spontaneously. Therefore, oral and maxillofacial surgeons are always careful about complications associated with the maxillary sinus. Furthermore, in general, otolaryngologists, leading physicians in paranasal sinus diseases, prefer to avoid direct contact with the sinus. Thus, an open transantral approach (the Caldwell-Luc operation) is rarely performed compared to less invasive endoscopic approaches, except for occasional situations [2]. Conversely, almost every dental implant practitioner interferes directly with the maxillary sinus or its neighboring parts in the alveolar bone and performs surgeries within close proximity to the antrum of Highmore. In particular, maxillary sinus augmentation has become one of the most popular dental procedures performed.

Maxillary sinus augmentation is a procedure that aims to increase the vertical bone height of the alveolar bone to allow placement of dental implants. For more than 30 years, the maxillary sinus augmentation procedure has been performed for implant-directed maxillary reconstruction [3]. There are various techniques, approaches, and materials used in this procedure. The purpose of this chapter is to review the essentials of maxillary sinus augmentation, clarify this procedure for otolaryngologists, explain its function, and describe the augmentation materials, techniques, and complications.

2. Assessment of alveolar bone quality for dental implants

Alveolar bone quantity and quality are the most important parameters primarily affecting the success of implant treatment. Sufficient bone support is the main requirement to gain osseointegration of implants. The buccolingual width is measured to predict the implant height. Allowing a bony distance in the apical region from the anatomical landmarks, such as the maxillary sinus, is also recommended. In addition to bone width and height, density is also critical for ensuring implant success [4]. It is important to place implants in locations with good primary stability, which cannot be acquired in regions with low bone density.

In addition to structure, a particular assessment of the available residual bone by morphological evaluation is crucial. Determinants of available bone might be listed as height, width, size, and incline [5]. Current advances in implant surface technologies revealed that implants of ~8–10-mm length provided long-term successful outcomes [6]. It is mandatory to have at least 1-mm buccal and lingual bony thickness adjacent to the implant [7]. For long-term success, implants should be inserted parallel to each other and to the adjacent teeth, to obtain the best stress distribution [8]. A detailed superstructure and prosthetic treatment plan should also be deliberated, considering occlusal forces, interocclusal distance, and interarch relations in the particular region [9]. Consequently, an alveolar bone assessment is performed not only to evaluate existing bone features and anatomy but also to estimate future dynamics in the overall treatment process, including prosthetic design, surrounding soft-tissue support, dental hygiene of the patient, and socioeconomic considerations, which provide long-term esthetics and functional outcomes of implant rehabilitation [10].

Both clinical and radiologic examinations are essential for treatment planning. The judgment of the clinician in treatment planning is paramount because each clinical case is unique. The medical history of the patient and a physical examination should be performed before treatment planning. History of nasal, sinus or maxillary surgery, chronic sinus/facial pain, acute upper respiratory infection, smoking habit, and chronic sinus disease are important to note. Panoramic X-ray imaging is generally used because it provides adequate information about the associated region. However, particular findings in panoramic imaging might lead the clinician to request further imaging methods, such as computed tomography (CT) or cone beam-computed tomography (CBCT). These techniques allow evaluating the exact amount of bone beneath the sinus floor, the sinus buccopalatal width, the presence of septa, and any preexisting sinus disease. Thus, based on a detailed CBCT examination, the necessary precautions can be taken, possible complications prevented, or surgery can be abandoned.

2.1. Anatomy

The maxillary sinus grows rapidly during childhood until it reaches the level of the floor of the nose. It may reach approximately 10 mm below the nasal floor [11]. The apexes of the maxillary premolars and molars have a close association with the inferior border of the maxillary sinus. The maxillary sinus extends to the premolar area at the anterior border and the roof is formed by the orbital floor.

The maxillary sinus volume increases continuously as a person ages, which is called pneumatization. It generally occurs in an inferior direction, frequently fasten with tooth extraction, such as loss of maxillary premolar or molars. It is reported that maxillary sinus pneumatization increases after tooth extractions [12]. Alveolar bone loss in the region creates a unique problem for implant placement following extraction. The pneumatization process can eventually result in extreme thinning of the alveolar bone and leave an inadequate amount of bone in the region assigned for dental implants. The vertical bone loss might occur only between the alveolar ridge crest and floor of the sinus, due to the resorption process following tooth extraction. It might also occur, while maintaining the level at the alveolar ridge crest with ongoing resorption under the sinus floor, due to increased osteoclast activity within the periosteum side of the Schneiderian membrane, or a combination of both occurrences. Additionally, low density of the posterior maxillary region might contribute to all these resorption processes, resulting in contour or dimensional changes (**Figure 1**). Considering interocclusal distance, prosthetic planning, predicted implant height and width, and also the density of the remaining bone are essential for successful prosthetic rehabilitation. The morphology of a bony defect is an important consideration in selecting an augmentation method. Sinus volume and the height of the semilunar hiatus define the maximum amount of elevation level of the membrane. An excessive amount of grafting material within the sinus may cause problems in sinus ventilation. The amount of sinus volume needed to raise the sinus floor is decided according to all these parameters.

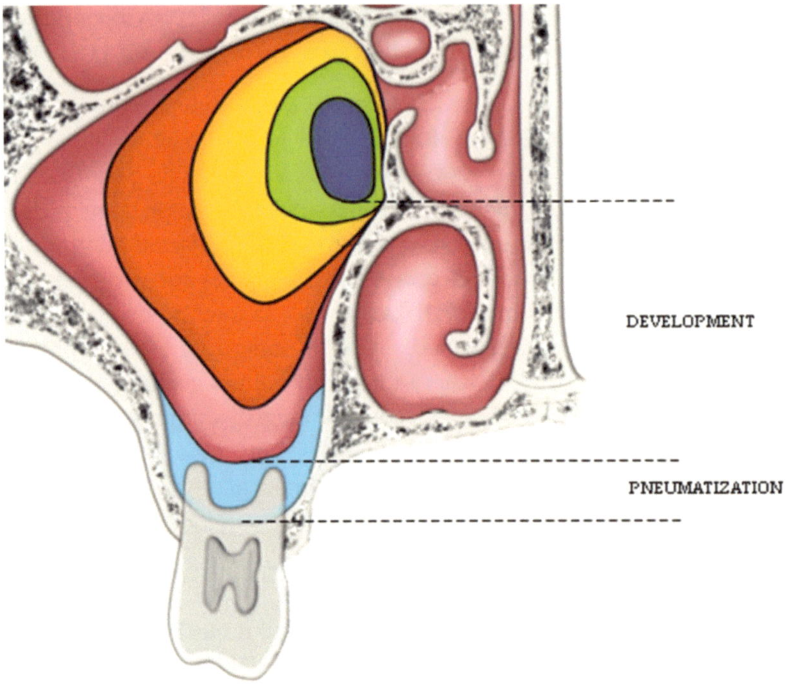

Figure 1. Pneumatization and development of maxillary sinus.

The Schneiderian membrane is a thin bilaminar mucoperiosteal membrane that lines the maxillary sinuses. One side of this membrane consists of epithelium, as per the remainder of the respiratory tract and nasal epithelium. The thin layer of pseudociliated stratified respiratory epithelium over the Schneiderian membrane establishes an important barrier for the protection and defense of the sinus cavity. The physiologic importance of the membrane cilia is to guide mucous discharge and debris toward the ostium so that in normal functioning, sinuses drainage is constantly maintained. Some conditions, such as allergic rhinitis, dysfunctional sinus cilia, or sinusitis might lead to local swelling and blockage of the ostium; therefore, subsequent blockage of outflowing mucous discharge can cause complications after sinus lifting. The membrane is ~0.8 mm thick. [13] The sinus mucosa is less vascular and thinner than nasal mucosa. Elevation of the membrane is a delicate procedure. Maintenance of its integrity is essential for normal functioning of the sinus after surgery. Perforation of the sinus membrane is the most common complication that has been reported since the earliest reports on the procedure. Some anatomical variations, particularly those concerning the septa, might trigger such perforation [14].

The maxillary sinus septa were first described by Underwood [15]. Numerous variations of the maxillary sinus septa are described in the literature, such as the partial perpendicular septa, the partial horizontal septa, and the complete septation of the maxillary sinus by a complete vertical septum. The height and setting of the septa are also important because the septa can hinder the preservation of the membrane. Sometimes, the sinus can be divided into two or more compartments. In such instances, the inversion of the bone plate and elevation of the Schneiderian membrane might be complicated. Septa generally arise between the areas of two adjacent teeth, and their formation might be promoted by the different phases of sinus pneumatization (**Figure 2**).

It is important to mention that a possible extraosseous anastomosis between the posterior superior alveolar artery and a terminal branch of the infraorbital artery might cause hemorrhage during flap elevation. An intraosseous anastomosis, by contrast, always occurs at a distance of 19–20 mm from the alveolar margin. If the intraosseous anastomosis is encountered during the preparation of the lateral bony window, hemorrhage might complicate the overall procedure.

2.2. Function

The aim of sinus floor elevation and augmentation is to create sufficient bone to house an implant with adequate stability. Pneumatization of the sinus results in an insufficient posterior maxillary alveolus. The adequate bone height and, thus, the moment when sinus floor elevation should be performed remain a controversial issue. Conversely, there are some other methods in which the sinus augmentation procedure is completely disregarded, such as using short implants, angulated implants, or distal cantilevers. All of these alternative methods are reported with long-term successful outcomes [16].

The requirement for maxillary sinus augmentation depends on the number of missing posterior teeth. If all premolars and molars are missing, it is more indispensable to perform sinus augmentation compared to a single missing molar or premolar tooth. The patient can choose to have a dental bridge restoration to replace a single missing tooth or two missing teeth. Moreover, patients missing all premolars and molars or do not have back teeth to support the bridge restoration might prefer a partial removable denture than maxillary sinus augmentation surgery [17].

The need for sinus augmentation is decided according to the size of the implant that is planned. Generally, implants are considered as short if it is smaller than 8 mm in height; therefore, it is expected that there should be >8 mm of subantral bone height to place the implants without sinus lifting. Various methods can be used while placing the implant in this region.

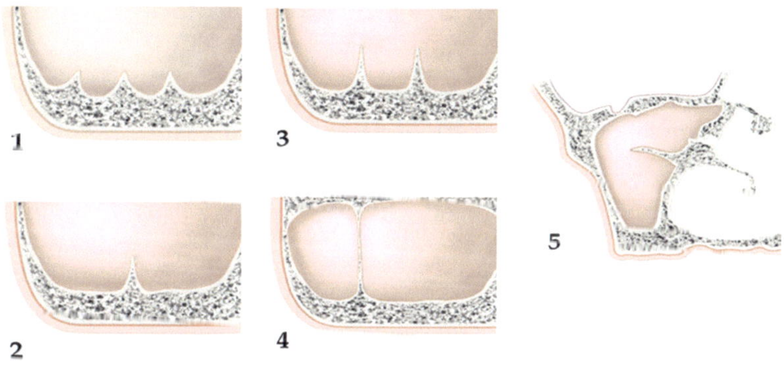

Figure 2. Possible variations of maxillary sinus septa. 1.Multiple septa , 2. Single septum , 3.Two basal septa , 4.Complete septum, 5.Partial horizontal septum.

The important point is to decide whether or not to interfere with the sinus when placing the implant. Essentially, it is important to have primary stabilization of the implant into the bone. For a successful osseointegration, the dental implant should be attached, or at least stay immobile, in the bone at the initial stages of the healing process. Based on these principles, the implant might be angulated to stay in the bone or shortened and thickened to increase the surrounding bony surface. However, it is well established that the implants should be placed parallel to each other in the long axis, as occurs in the natural roots.

2.3. Contraindication

The aim of maxillary sinus augmentation surgery is to place dental implants. Therefore, some contraindications with implant surgery are valid for sinus augmentation. Soft- and hard-tissue support of a predicted dental implant should be established before placement of a dental implant. Local or systemic conditions can compromise the bone healing and the osseointegration. Before planning sinus augmentation for dental implants, the patient's usual healing should be questioned and the sinus should be evaluated in detail. A sinus infection can directly affect the success of the sinus-lifting procedure. During the delicate lifting phase or following surgery, inflammatory fluid in the sinus can easily infiltrate to the augmented site and distract graft healing. Therefore, patients with acute sinus inflammation should be treated for their sinus disease. Smoking and chronic sinusitis can increase the risks associated with the sinus augmentation procedure. In smokers, the sinus membrane can be considerably thin and fragile, which contribute to ready laceration of the membrane during elevation. By contrast, chronic sinusitis and allergies may result in a thick membrane, which can also complicate membrane elevation. Any other finding associated with maxillary sinus disease requires consultation with an otolaryngologist during preoperative planning [18].

Uncontrolled diabetes, neoplasm, radiotherapy, or chemotherapy can also be considered contraindications to sinus augmentation for dental implants. Additionally, previous sinus surgeries or Le Fort I osteotomy may also be a contraindication because of the scar formation after surgery [19].

3. Graft materials used in maxillary sinus augmentation

Various materials have been used to graft the floor of the sinus and achieve the desired bone height. Grafting materials can be categorized based on their source, as autograft, xenograft, allograft, and alloplastic. These different types of grafting materials may be used alone or in any combination. Bone grafts heal by three different mechanisms: osteogenesis, osteoinduction, and osteoconduction. Osteogenesis is the ability to produce new bone. Osteoinduction is the process of stimulating osteogenesis. Finally, osteoconduction is the ability of a material to support the growth of bone over its surface. Grafting materials mostly use the mechanism of osteoconductivity to provide biomechanical support, stabilize the components during the healing phase, and establish the scaffold for new bone formation. The best graft healing should possess most of these mechanisms.

An autograft is considered as the golden standard for maxillary sinus augmentation. It has osteogenic, osteoinductive, and osteoconductive features. Furthermore, it has the best biocompatibility feature. However, it also has the disadvantage of donor-site morbidity. Extraoral or intraoral donor sites constitute a secondary surgical site and the risk of associated complications. They also have the highest rate of resorption. Autografts can be harvested from multiple sites. The amount of required bone amount is the main determinant for choosing the harvesting site. Donor-site morbidity and patient's preferences are the other important factors to consider when choosing the harvesting site. Intraoral mandibular symphysis, mandibular ramus, and tuberosity can present a moderate to small amount of bone for this procedure. Additional bone can be provided from any other intraoral-harvesting site or by adding some other source of ready-to-use graft material, such as xenograft or allograft if required. Autografts might be particulated using a bone mill or a bone grinder to spread the material out in the bony space or extend the volume. Particulated grafts can facilitate vascular infiltration, angiogenesis, bone matrix formation, and, thus, better healing. A mixture of the particulated bone chips with blood or platelet-rich fibrin can also enhance better bone matrix organization.

If additional autograft is needed or bilateral sinus augmentation is required or an additional onlay grafting is necessary, extraoral-harvesting sites, which present a significant amount of bone (~50 ml), can be used. Extraoral-harvesting sites can be ranked as providing the most amount of bone to relatively less: posterior ilium, anterior ilium, calvarium, and tibia. As expected, because of donor-site morbidity and requirement for more advanced surgeries, extraoral harvesting is not generally preferred by the patients. The calvarium has never been a priority harvesting site for a relatively simple bone augmentation surgery to place a dental implant. However, when other alternatives have failed and most of the donor sites had been attempted without success, it stands as an option. Complications at the donor sites after autogenous bone harvesting include infection, dental injury, pain, sensory disturbances, gait disturbance, and hernia, for example.

Allogeneic graft materials are also biocompatible and have some osteoconductive potential. They originate from humans and are acquired from tissue banks. However, the risk of disease transmission and high resorption rate are the main disadvantages of these graft materials. The mineralized form of these grafts is not preferred due to the slow bone formation rate, while demineralized forms are mostly preferred due to their bone morphogenic protein ingredients and associated osteoconductive feature. Alloplastic graft materials are made from hydroxyapatite, calcium phosphates, and bioactive glass. Also, they have a lower rate of resorption compared to autologous grafts. Xenografts are derived from a donor of a species different than the recipient. Deproteinized bovine bone is widely used in sinus augmentation surgery due to good osteoconductivity and can be used alone, or in combination with, other grafting materials.

All graft materials have different healing times, from 4 to 10 months. The resorption rate of the graft material is an important parameter in the sinus augmentation procedure because the volume of the graft will decrease if the material resorbs quickly. Waiting for the formation of qualified bone is critical to place the implant in the vital bone. Placement of implants can be performed earlier in such materials compared to non-resorbable materials. Alloplastic graft materials, calcium sulfate, and beta-tricalcium phosphate resorb quickly, while bioglass resorbs considerably more slowly. Therefore, deciding the most appropriate time to place the implant according to the properties of the graft material is necessary. Autogenous bone and xenografts are reported to produce the most predictable and best results in sinus augmentation [20].

Knowing the features of the grafting material used plays a major role in the overall outcome and success of the grafting procedure. The posterior maxillary region and sinus membrane are rich in vasculature; therefore, grafting materials placed in these regions will have a rich blood supply. This regional advantage also enhances the osteoblastic activity of the augmented site. The importance of the membrane in the sinus-lift procedure should not be underestimated. It is reported that the Schneiderian membrane has the feature of inducing and increasing osteoprogenitor cells [21]. Various techniques are used to create a bony space for implant placement while maintaining the membrane intact to allow for graft nutrition and a barrier from the maxillary sinus cavity. Obtaining successful outcomes depends on multiple factors. Besides the unique anatomical features of every case, the surgeon's experience and the method used for augmentation are pivotal. Selecting the most proper technique for every individual case and applying sound surgical techniques at the appropriate surgical site are mandatory to obtain long-term successful outcomes.

4. Grafting techniques

Maxillary sinus lifting can be performed directly with lateral antrostomy under direct visualization or indirectly with the transalveolar approach. The amount of residual maxillary alveolar bone defines which approach to be used for sinus augmentation. Bone height below the sinus, alveolar bone width, and sinus anatomy should be assessed in detail, and CBCT can assist in providing accurate measurements. The indirect technique is used when the required augmentation height is 3 mm or less [22].

4.1. Direct technique

As first demonstrated by Tatum [23], the direct technique is performed with direct visualization of the sinus membrane. Initially, a midcrestal or palatally positioned incision is made in the mesiodistal direction along the length of the alveolar crest. Anterior- and posterior-releasing incisions are made. The incision should extend at least one tooth beyond the planned side. Adequate surgical exposure and visualization are directly related to the size of the incision. A full-thickness mucoperiosteal flap with a trapezoid base is elevated while maintaining periosteal integrity. The mucoperiosteal flap elevation should be performed carefully and start from the midcrest (i.e., more palatal region) to avoid exposure of the grafting area in the event of wound dehiscence. The size of the incision directly affects the manipulation during surgery, the size of the osteotomy, augmentation stage, and placement of the implant. Therefore, this stage should not be underestimated.

The superoinferior and anteroposterior borders of the lateral window are determined by the sinus volume, which is preoperatively examined by radiography. After mucoperiosteal flap elevation, most of the time shadow of the sinus space can be distinguished intraoperatively.

The inferior border of the lateral bony window should be 2–5 mm superior to the sinus floor, to prevent tearing of the sinus membrane and difficulty during infracturing. The anterior border is determined by the mesial extent of the sinus to the point that the sinus curette can extend and be manipulated for elevation, whereas the distal border determines the most posteriorly planned implant's location. The shape of the osteotomy window can be rectangular or oval and outlined with a size of ~10 × 20 mm. The size of the window can increase or decrease, according to the size of the planned region that needs augmentation for implant placement. In some instances, it is necessary to prepare two openings, due to the presence of septa, to prevent laceration of the membrane (**Figure 3**) [24, 25].

The osteotomy starts by outlining the lateral window with a round bur until a bluish hue is visible along the outline. The osteotomy continues by connecting the holes. The center native bone window can either remain in place or be removed for replacement after the augmentation. However, when the bony window is small, the entire center part can be readily discarded during preparation. Finally, sharp edges and corners should be rounded to prevent membrane perforation during elevation [26].

There are various techniques available to perform a lateral sinus wall osteotomy. Different methods and various bur types or instruments exist to prevent tearing of the sinus mucosa. Traditional carbide or diamond burs are used for access preparations. Alternatively, a diamond-studded concave bur is used to prevent perforation during osteotomy. In addition, piezosurgery is an ultrasonic method, advised for its selective osteotomy with membrane preservation. The piezoelectric surgery systems have been designed to use a specific power, which allows the osteotomies to be made in thick and compact cortical bone. The real advantage of piezosurgery is that it does not cut soft tissue and helps to reduce the chance of perforating the membrane. It can also be used to detach the sinus membrane from the bone before elevation. Piezosurgery can be most useful in the instances involving considerable cortical bone and thin membranes. However, regardless of the method or instrument used, the sinus membrane is extremely fine and thin; thus, it can easily rupture when treated roughly or pressed during an osteotomy. Hence, clinicians should always be gentle during osteotomy and lifting [27, 28].

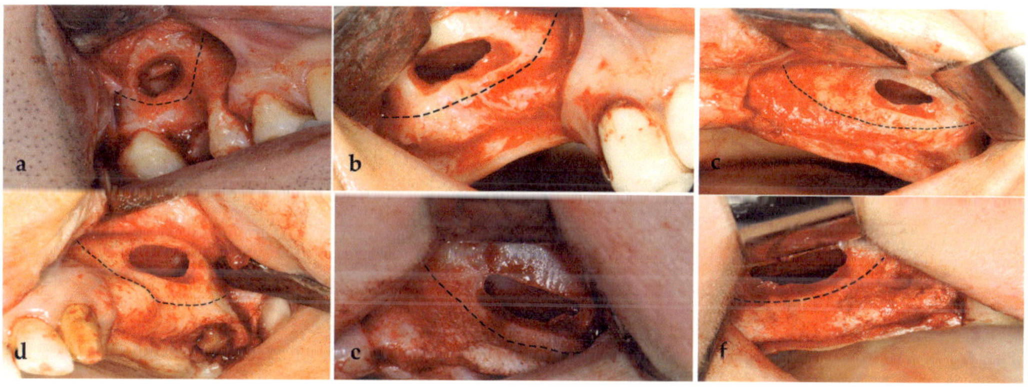

Figure 3. Various lateral windows to approach maxillary sinus membrane.

Once the sinus membrane starts to be detached from the corners and edges, the elevation can be performed using broad-based freers or curettes. Complete detachment of the membrane from all surfaces should be performed slowly and never lose bone contact. Before pushing the membrane in an upward direction, it should be assured that the membrane is separated from the bone. It is important to do this without excessive pressure. This releasing and detachment process is implemented until reaching the level of intended height. The most common mistake during this step is not to extend the medial side of the sinus, potentially leading to sinus perforation, while putting bone graft material due to the applied insertion pressure or to membrane damage when drilling the implant site [22].

In the one-stage protocol, when there is sufficient bone to support primary implant stability, which is about 5 mm in height, implant-site preparation is made according to the implant company's recommendation. During drilling, care should be taken not to harm the membrane with the tip of the implant drill [29]. In the two-stage protocol, the prepared graft material is placed by pieces into the drilled hole, followed by a 6-month wait. The particulated bone graft is then inserted into the bony floor space. The graft particles should reach the farthest distance, loosely placed, dispersed homogeneously, and should not be overpacked. After the bone is placed in the sinus, the mucoperiosteal flap is positioned and primary closure is achieved (**Figure 4**) [30].

4.2. Indirect technique

Developed by Summers in 1994, the indirect technique consists of a crestal incision, preparation of the bone, and elevation of the sinus by several millimeters [31]. The transalveolar sinus-lift technique is more conservative than the open approach. The sinus membrane is not directly instrumented. Also, the sinus cavity is not directly visualized and membrane perforations are more difficult to determine. This technique can be used when there is at least 5–6 mm of alveolar bone. A 4–8-mm bone height gain is achieved by using this technique. The augmentation procedure and implant-site preparation are performed simultaneously. However, there is an upper limit of intrusion regarding the amount of bone and tensile strength of the sinus mucosa because of the pushing without detachment. In this technique, the implant space is prepared not only by compacting the bone apically and elevating the sinus but also by compacting the bone laterally by using osteotomes of progressively increasing diameter [32, 33].

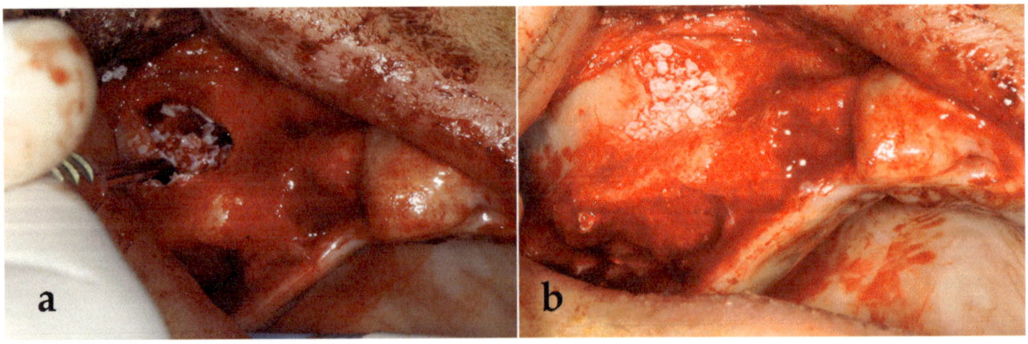

Figure 4. Insertion of bone graft into the bony space under the schneiderian membrane.

Once a full-thickness mucoperiosteal flap has been elevated, a marking drill is used to identify the exact place of the implant. A pilot drill (1-mm diameter) is used only to an initial depth of a few millimeters. It should be about 2 mm away from the sinus floor. Next, a mallet is used to drive the osteotomes. The first osteotome fractures the cortical border of the maxillary sinus floor. A gradual increase in the depth decreases the risk of membrane tear. Larger osteotomes are used, respectively, to the final implant depth until the planned implant width. The final osteotome should have a smaller diameter than the planned implant diameter, to obtain initial implant stability. For implantation in low-density bone, it might be considered to add some bone graft below the implant because of the lack of compressed bone. The mucoperiosteal flap is repositioned and primary closure is achieved after the implant placement [22, 26].

There are some other techniques for maxillary sinus augmentation surgery. For example, the balloon technique is an indirect sinus elevation method [34], performed with application of a balloon via a transcrestal approach that elevates the sinus membrane while the balloon inflates. Another method used does not involve a bone graft. In this technique, there must be some vertical bone height for holding the implant in a stable position (at least 5 mm). The sinus membrane is elevated traditionally via a lateral antrostomy approach; then, the implant is placed without any bone graft. The implant stands under the elevated sinus floor and elevated sinus membrane creates a tenting effect over the implant. The osteoprogenitor potential of the sinus membrane is believed to produce a bony support around the apical portion of the implant in time. This technique is called graftless lateral sinus floor elevation [35, 36].

5. Postoperative instructions after sinus augmentation surgery

There are several things that the patient should be informed about after surgery. Initially, routine postoperative instructions for oral-surgical procedures should be communicated, such as the application of ice and pressure to the site, elevation of the head, and rest. Additionally, patients should be instructed about sinus precautions, which are avoiding anything that can cause sudden pressure changes in the sinus, such as nose blowing with nostrils pinched closed and sneezing with a closed mouth. If there is an increase in pressure in the sinus, perforations and displacement of the particulate graft are possible and it prevents graft maturation and healing [26, 37]. In addition, the patient should be advised to take medications (such as anti-inflammatory drugs, antibiotics, and nasal decongestants) as prescribed by the surgeon.

6. Complications

The most frequently encountered surgical complication is perforation of the sinus membrane. It occurs particularly in the direct technique due to vigorous elevation, a thin membrane, sharp edges and ridges, and septated or irregular topography of the sinus. If the perforation is missed or not properly sealed, extravasation of the particulate graft into the maxillary sinus might predispose the patient to an infection or result in poor graft retention in the area. Management of this complication is made according to the size of the perforation [14]. Small perforations are relocated in an area where the elevated mucosa folds together. In such instances, there is no need for further management. For larger perforations, attempts should be made to isolate and cover the gap with a resorbable membrane, to prevent loss of the graft into the sinus. If the perforation is sufficiently large that it cannot be covered by a resorbable membrane, the procedure is abandoned and a second surgery is considered after 2 months. Sinus perforations also increase the rates of postoperative sinusitis, infection, and graft failure [38].

The other reported complication of the sinus-lifting procedure is significant bleeding from the posterior superior alveolar artery. In some patients, arterial anastomoses can superficially exist on the lateral sinus wall. The location of the posterior superior alveolar artery should be considered before every surgery. Precautions must be taken to avoid massive bleeding and the trajectory of this artery should be considered after detailed CBCT examination. This artery might be encountered during a lateral wall osteotomy and compromise visibility of the surgical field, which can increase the possibility of membrane perforation and complicate placement of the graft. Therefore, the procedure may need to be stopped until the bleeding is controlled [39].

Maxillary septa are another issue that can complicate the sinus augmentation procedure. Their potential existence should be considered and necessary precautions should be taken. It is difficult or even impossible to separate the sinus membrane from septa without a tear. Preoperative evaluation with CBCT is useful to approach sinus septa while performing a lateral antrostomy. Most septa are located in the middle region of the antrum. Different methods, such as increasing the size of the bony window or preparing more than one lateral window, are available to overcome this issue [40].

Postoperative infection is another unwanted complication after maxillary sinus augmentation. In a case of infection spreading into the sinus, the infected graft material should be removed. Systemic antibiotics are to be adjusted accordingly. Graft failure is expected in these cases. It may also be necessary to remove the grafted material to clear the infection [18]. Patient selection, treatment planning, and the appropriate sinus augmentation technique are essential to minimize the risk of complications.

Author details

Gökhan Göçmen* and Yasar Özkan

*Address all correspondence to: gocmengokhan@hotmail.com

Department of Oral and Maxillofacial Surgery, Faculty of Dentistry, Marmara University, Istanbul, Turkey

References

[1] Anzalone JV, Vastardis S. Oroantral communication as an osteotome sinus elevation complication. Journal of Oral Implantology. 2010;**36**:231–237. DOI: 10.1563/AAID-JOI-D-09-00026

[2] Macbeth R. Caldwell, Luc, and their operation. Laryngoscope. 1971;**81**:1652–1657. DOI: 10.1288/00005537-197110000-00011

[3] Mohan N, Wolf J, Dym H. Maxillary sinus augmentation. Dental Clinics of North America. 2015;**59**:375–388. DOI: 10.1016/j.cden.2014.10.001

[4] Drage NA, Palmer RM, Blake G, Wilson R, Crane F, Fogelman I. A comparison of bone mineral density in the spine, hip and jaws of edentulous subjects. Clinical Oral Implants Research. 2007;**18**:496–500. DOI: 10.1111/j.1600-0501.2007.01379.x

[5] Lundgren S, Cricchio G, Hallman M, Jungner M, Rasmusson L, Sennerby L. Sinus floor elevation procedures to enable implant placement and integration: techniques, biological aspects and clinical outcomes. Periodontology 2000. 2017;**73**:103–120. DOI: 10.1111/prd.12165

[6] Thor A, Sennerby L, Hirsch JM, Rasmusson L. Bone formation at the maxillary sinus floor following simultaneous elevation of the mucosal lining and implant installation without graft material: An evaluation of 20 patients treated with 44 Astra Tech implants. Journal of Oral & Maxillofacial Surgery. 2007;**65**:64–72. DOI: 10.1016/j.joms.2006.10.047

[7] Temmerman A, Keestra JA, Coucke W, Teughels W, Quirynen M. The outcome of oral implants placed in bone with limited bucco-oral dimensions: A 3-year follow-up study. Journal of Clinical Periodontology. 2015;**42**:311–318. DOI: 10.1111/jcpe.12376

[8] Ramaglia L, Toti P, Sbordone C, Guidetti F, Martuscelli R, Sbordone L. Implant angulation: 2-year retrospective analysis on the influence of dental implant angle insertion on marginal bone resorption in maxillary and mandibular osseous onlay grafts. Clinical Oral Investigation. 2015;**19**:769–779. DOI: 10.1007/s00784-014-1275-5

[9] Blanes RJ, Bernard JP, Blanes ZM, Belser UC. A 10-year prospective study of ITI dental implants placed in the posterior region. II: Influence of the crown-to-implant ratio and different prosthetic treatment modalities on crestal bone loss. Clinical Oral Implants Research. 2007;**18**:707–714. DOI: 10.1111/j.1600-0501.2006.01307.x

[10] Clark D, Levin L. Dental implant management and maintenance: How to improve long-term implant success? Quintessence International. 2016;**47**:417–423. DOI: 10.3290/j.qi.a35870

[11] Lawson W, Patel ZM, Lin FY. The development and pathologic processes that influence maxillary sinus pneumatization. Anatomical Record (Hoboken). 2008;**291**:1554–1563. DOI: 10.1002/ar.20774

[12] Sharan A, Madjar D. Maxillary sinus pneumatization following extractions: A radiographic study. International Journal of Oral & Maxillofacial Implants. 2008;**23**:48–56

[13] Makary C, Rebaudi A, Menhall A, Naaman N. Changes in sinus membrane thickness after lateral sinus floor elevation: A radiographic study. International Journal of Oral & Maxillofacial Implants. 2016;**31**:331–337. DOI: 10.11607/jomi.4108

[14] Monje A, Monje-Gil F, Burgueno M, Gonzalez-Garcia R, Galindo-Moreno P, Wang HL. Incidence of and factors associated with sinus membrane perforation during maxillary sinus augmentation using the reamer drilling approach: A double-center case series. International Journal of Periodontics & Restorative Dentistry. 2016;**36**:549–556. DOI: 10.11607/prd.2525

[15] Underwood AS. An inquiry into the anatomy and pathology of the maxillary sinus. Journal of Anatomical Physiology. 1910;**44**:354–369

[16] Jain N, Gulati M, Garg M, Pathak C. Short implants: New horizon in implant dentistry. Journal of Clinical and Diagnostic Research. 2016;**10**:ZE14–ZE17. DOI: 10.7860/JCDR/2016/21838.8550

[17] Pieri F, Caselli E, Forlivesi C, Corinaldesi G. Rehabilitation of the atrophic posterior maxilla using splinted short implants or sinus augmentation with standard-length implants: A retrospective cohort study. International Journal of Oral & Maxillofacial Implants. 2016;**31**:1179–1188. DOI: 10.11607/jomi.4370

[18] Moreno Vazquez JC, Gonzalez de Rivera AS, Gil HS, Mifsut RS. Complication rate in 200 consecutive sinus lift procedures: Guidelines for prevention and treatment. Journal of Oral & Maxillofacial Surgery. 2014;**72**:892–901. DOI: 10.1016/j.joms.2013.11.023

[19] Schwarz L, Schiebel V, Hof M, Ulm C, Watzek G, Pommer B. Risk factors of membrane perforation and postoperative complications in sinus floor elevation surgery: Review of 407 augmentation procedures. Journal of Oral & Maxillofacial Surgery. 2015;**73**:1275–1282. DOI: 10.1016/j.joms.2015.01.039

[20] Araujo DB, de Jesus Campos E, Oliveira MA, Lima MJ, Martins GB, Araujo RP. Surgical elevation of bilateral maxillary sinus floor with a combination of autogenous bone and lyophilized bovine bone. The Journal of Contemporary and Dental Practice. 2013;**14**:445–450

[21] Srouji S, Ben-David D, Lotan R, Riminucci M, Livne E, Bianco P. The innate osteogenic potential of the maxillary sinus (Schneiderian) membrane: An ectopic tissue transplant model simulating sinus lifting. International Journal of Oral & Maxillofacial Surgery. 2010;**39**:793–801. DOI: 10.1016/j.ijom.2010.03.009

[22] Carrao V, DeMatteis I. Maxillary sinus bone augmentation techniques. Oral & Maxillofacial Surgery Clinics of North America. 2015;**27**:245–253. DOI: 10.1016/j.coms.2015.01.001

[23] Tatum H, Jr. Maxillary and sinus implant reconstructions. Dental Clinics of North America. 1986;**30**:207–229

[24] Romanos GE. Window preparation for sinus lift procedures: A simplified technique. Implant Dentistry. 2008;**17**:377–381. DOI: 10.1097/ID.0b013e31818c65f6

[25] Vercellotti T, De Paoli S, Nevins M. The piezoelectric bony window osteotomy and sinus membrane elevation: Introduction of a new technique for simplification of the sinus augmentation procedure. International Journal of Periodontics & Restorative Dentistry. 2001;**21**:561–567

[26] Stern A, Green J. Sinus lift procedures: An overview of current techniques. Dental Clinics of North America. 2012;**56**:219–233. DOI: x. 10.1016/j.cden.2011.09.003

[27] Kuhl S, Kirmeier R, Platzer S, Bianco N, Jakse N, Payer M. Transcrestal maxillary sinus augmentation: Summers' versus a piezoelectric technique – an experimental cadaver study. ClinicalOral Implants Research. 2016;**27**:126–129. DOI: 10.1111/clr.12546

[28] Cassetta M, Ricci L, Iezzi G, Calasso S, Piattelli A, Perrotti V. Use of piezosurgery during maxillary sinus elevation: Clinical results of 40 consecutive cases. International Journal of Periodontics & Restorative Dentistry. 2012;**32**:e182–e188

[29] Kahnberg KE, Ekestubbe A, Grondahl K, Nilsson P, Hirsch JM. Sinus lifting procedure. I. One-stage surgery with bone transplant and implants. Clinical Oral Implants Research. 2001;**12**:479–487

[30] Galindo-Moreno P, Avila G, Fernandez-Barbero JE, Aguilar M, Sanchez-Fernandez E, Cutando A, et al. Evaluation of sinus floor elevation using a composite bone graft mixture. Clinical Oral Implants Research. 2007;**18**:376–382. DOI: 10.1111/j.1600-0501.2007.01337.x

[31] Summers RB. A new concept in maxillary implant surgery: The osteotome technique. Compendium. 1994;**15**:152 (154–156, 158 passim; quiz 162)

[32] Agamy EM, Niedermeier W. Indirect sinus floor elevation for osseointegrated prostheses. A 10-year prospective study. Journal of Oral Implantology. 2010;**36**:113–121. DOI: 10.1563/AAID-JOI-D-09-00085

[33] Draenert GF, Eisenmenger W. A new technique for the transcrestal sinus floor elevation and alveolar ridge augmentation with press-fit bone cylinders: a technical note. Journal of Craniomaxillofacial Surgery. 2007;**35**:201–206. DOI: 10.1016/j.jcms.2007.02.005

[34] Kotsakis GA, Mazor Z. A simplified approach to the minimally invasive antral membrane elevation technique utilizing a viscoelastic medium for hydraulic sinus floor elevation. Oral and Maxillofacial Surgery. 2015;**19**:97–101. DOI: 10.1007/s10006-014-0473-2

[35] Kosinski TF. Sinus tenting for posterior maxillary implant placement. Dentistry Today. 2014;**33**:58–61

[36] Falah M, Sohn DS, Srouji S. Graftless sinus augmentation with simultaneous dental implant placement: clinical results and biological perspectives. International Journal of Oral and Maxillofacial Surgery. 2016;**45**:1147–1153. DOI: 10.1016/j.ijom.2016.05.006

[37] Del Fabbro M, Corbella S, Ceresoli V, Ceci C, Taschieri S. Plasma rich in growth factors improves patients' postoperative quality of life in maxillary sinus floor augmentation: Preliminary results of a randomized clinical study. Clinical Implant Dentistry and Related Research. 2015;**17**:708–716. DOI: 10.1111/cid.12171

[38] Shiffler K, Lee D, Aghaloo T, Moy PK, Pi-Anfruns J. Sinus membrane perforations and the incidence of complications: A retrospective study from a residency program. Oral Surgery, Oral Medicine, Oral Pathology, Oral Radiology. 2015;**120**:10–14. DOI: 10.1016/j.oooo.2015.02.477

[39] Varela-Centelles P, Loira-Gago M, Gonzalez-Mosquera A, Seoane-Romero JM, Garcia-Martin JM, Seoane J. Distance of the alveolar antral artery from the alveolar crest. Related factors and surgical considerations in sinus floor elevation. Medicina Oral, Patologia Oral Y Cirugia Bucal. 2016;**21**:e758–e765

[40] Al-Dajani M. Incidence, risk factors, and complications of schneiderian membrane perforation in sinus lift surgery: A meta-analysis. Implant Dentistry. 2016;**25**:409–415. DOI: 10.1097/ID.0000000000000411

Section 3

Radiological Imaging

Chapter 3

CBCT Imaging of Paranasal Sinuses and Variations

Kaan Orhan, Secil Aksoy and Ulas Oz

Additional information is available at the end of the chapter

http://dx.doi.org/10.5772/intechopen.69090

Abstract

Paranasal sinuses located in the bones surrounding the nasal cavity are called maxillary, ethmoid, frontal and sphenoid sinuses. In relation with their location, these sinuses contribute to the development of the facial structures, jaws and upper airway. During the developmental process of the paranasal sinuses, anatomic variations can occur in consequence of intra and extramural migration of the ethmoid air cells, overpneumatization or hypoplasia of the sinuses and bulging of the neurovascular structures to the sinuses. Some of these anatomic variations may affect the drainage pathways, pave the way for chronic infections and cause difficulties when performing paranasal sinuses surgery. Therefore, the aim of this chapter was to examine the paranasal sinus anatomic variations with cone beam computed tomography (CBCT).

Keywords: cone beam computed tomography, paranasal sinuses, anatomic variations

1. Introduction

Paranasal sinuses are located in the bones surrounding the nasal cavity; and they are called according to anatomical relations such as maxillary, ethmoid, frontal and sphenoid sinuses. The sinuses develop mostly after birth, and their degree of development varies greatly. It is controversial that paranasal sinuses have an aid to facial growth and development or persist as residual remnants of an evolutionary structure found in an additional role as an adjunct to the nasal cavity [1 5]. There are numerous results explaining the function of paranasal sinuses.

In relation with their location, these sinuses contribute to the development of the facial structures, jaws, upper airway, some degree of warmth and humidification to inspired air, thermal isolation, resonance of voice, weight of the skull and expansion of olfactory surfaces.

The paranasal sinuses can act to improve nasal function; they improve the production of nitric oxide and in aiding the immune defences of the nasal cavity [1]. Besides, the sinuses can show adaptability to environmental stress in relation to human facial morphology, for example, human paranasal sinuses have been shown to have higher volumes in individuals living in warmer climates [2, 3].

Additionally, there are findings relating the paranasal sinuses with vascular thermal mechanism. The vascular mechanism in which the arterial blood destined for the brain is cooled by venous blood returning from the evaporating surfaces of the head is called the carotid rete [4]. However, in terms of missing the selective brain cooling mechanism temporarily or permanently, a vascular structure that facilitates counter-current heat exchange is located at the base of the skull in some mammals. In case of lacking a vascular mechanism or an aid to the selective brain cooling system, larger paranasal sinuses and also broader nasal cavity would be providing more evaporating surfaces; such variations have been shown in individuals, especially living in hot climates [4].

Paranasal sinuses may assure harmony in facial growth and make the skull lighter. They also can be seen as a protector of the brain. In prenatal growth and development, the facial cranium distinctly retracts, the maxillary sinus is enlarged because of the new osteogenic activity for erupting molar teeth. During embryogenic life, the functions of the sinuses such as air conditioning progress in harmony with the change in the dental arch and the enlargement of the masticatory muscles.

In addition, the mucociliary apparatus has an important role in maintaining the integrity of the nasal airway and paranasal sinuses as well as that of the rest of the respiratory tract, that is, mucociliary transport relies not only on coordinated ciliary activity but also on mucus and its specific rheological properties.

2. Imaging techniques of paranasal sinuses

2.1. Conventional X rays

The conventional imaging techniques have included Water's (occipitomental view), Caldwell (occipitofrontal view), lateral (cephalometric), basal and oblique and submentovertex radiographies for the sinuses.

Sinus X rays are still frequently used in the evaluation of paranasal sinuses. The conventional diagnostic tools of two-dimensional X rays have shown various advantages such as low amount of radiation doses, simple and quick, noninvasive and low-cost advantages. According to recent studies, a low-dose high-resolution three-dimensional scans might be given more accurate diagnostic data for certain conditions such as surgical intervention, anatomic variations and nasal and osteomeatal unit evaluation. However, appearance of new digital two-dimensional systems with numerous features of image enhancement, in addition to the mentioned advantages, might represent digital two-dimensional radiography as a simple and acceptable modality in this field [5].

The Water's view is also known as the occipitomental view, where the Xray beam is angled at 37° to the canthomeatal line. The radiographic plate is placed positioning towards the face and perpendicular to the midsagittal plane. It is commonly used to view of maxillary sinuses.

Lateral X-ray images show the osteogenic border of maxillary, sphenoid and frontal sinuses. It specially is used to survey the skull and facial bones for evidence of disease, trauma and developmental anomalies in orthodontics. Lateral cephalograms is also used for assessing facial growth.

Caldwell's view projects the osteogenic border of frontal sinus well. It has also included excellent capability in illustrating opasified frontal sinuses and ethmoidal air cells as well as nasal septum deviation [5].

Submentovertex view often is used for evaluating fractures and displacement of fractured zygomatic arch. However, this view is contraindicated with the cases suspected for spinal injury. On the other hand, it reveals the position of the condyles, sphenoid sinus, and the lateral wall of maxillary sinuses, which is an obvious advantage of visualizing of paranasal sinuses' air and fluid levels for sphenoid sinus. But, the view could be ineffective to reveal the degree of chronic inflammatory diseases especially for ethmoid sinuses [6]. Yet some findings such as opacification of the sphenoid sinus in mucocele, the radiographic identification is usually possible [7]. Such inconstancies emphasize the need for more detailed tomography [5–7].

2.2. Computed tomography

Computed tomography (CT) is currently the modality of choice in the evaluation of paranasal sinuses. A variety of CT scans such as conventional and/or cone beam CT techniques offer certain advantages and disadvantages even in comparison with other imaging techniques. Therefore, a primary concern to the clinician evaluating the paranasal sinuses should be conceiving an effective methodology [6–8].

CT imaging of the sinuses has been acquired in the axial, antero-posterior, and coronal planes as well as three-dimensional visual images using contiguous scans [8]. Either two-dimensional or three-dimensional usage of CT scans brings various advantages such as displaying bone and soft tissue anatomy and extent of diseases related with paranasal sinuses and around the paranasal sinuses [6–8]. In contrast, the conventional X-ray imaging methods, CT scans, can guide clearly visualization of the sinus anatomy, ostiomeatal channels, which is extremely useful in the pre-operative planning and in post-operative follow-up in cases of surgical interventions. Thus, the combination of CT scans with additional imaging methods such as functional endoscopy will bring significant advantage to treat particular cases more effectively, facilitating reduced morbidity and complications.

It is well stated that current multi-slice multi-channel CT scanners can acquire slices as thin as 0.5-mm images in any desired plane [6]. In some special conditions, such as lack of availability of multi-channel CT scan, scanning might be routinely finalized with contiguous 3-mm-thick images [6]. Although the diagnostic quality of CT scanning is accepted as sufficient, the radiation dose may be controversial [7, 8]. Therefore, numerous considerable reduction techniques in radiation exposure alternatives have been the most challenging issue for the manufacturer. Recently, cone beam computed tomography (CBCT) was introduced for dental and maxillofacial imaging [9]. CBCT has several advantages over traditional CT, including lower radiation dose, higher image resolution and lower cost of machine [10]. CBCT scans can be as thin as 0.125 mm, compared to 0.5–3 mm for CT.

2.3. Cone beam computed tomography

CBCT was first described in 1980 and was first applied to dentomaxillofacial radiology in 1998 [11, 12]. CBCT is accepted as one of the pioneering tool assessing paranasal sinuses by dentists, maxillofacial radiologists and otolaryngologists [11]. The technique has several advantages as mentioned above such as higher resolution and lower radiation doses.

3. Variations of paranasal sinuses

During the developmental process of the paranasal sinuses, ethmoid sinuses have a strategic central position. Especially, extramural and intramural expansion of the ethmoid cells causes highly variable anatomy in the nasal complex [13]. These anatomic variations may contribute to the occurrence of the paranasal sinus disease or cause operative complications when performing sinus surgery. While some of the anatomic variations such as concha bullosa, agger nasi cell (ANC), nasal septum deviation, pneumatization of the uncinate process and Haller's cell compromise already narrow the drainage pathways and produce obstruction in the osteomeatal unit (OMU) and thereby recurrent sinusitis [14], others from the onodi cell, protrusion of the internal carotid artery (ICA), optic nerve (ON), vidian canal (VC) and maxillary nerve (MN) to the sphenoid sinus can cause complications such as fatal bleeding, blindness and neurologic sequelae [15]. Consequently, it is necessary to determine the anatomy and the variations of the sinuses, particularly when the patient needs functional endoscopic sinus surgery (FESS).

3.1. Agger nasi cell

Embryologically, the lateral nasal wall has five foetal ridges and six furrows. Each ridge has an ascending and descending part. While some of the ridges and furrows disappear or fuse, some of them compromise the nasal concha. No concha develops from the first ethmoturbinal, but the remnant of the ascending portion forms the ANC [16, 17].

Extramural migration of the anterior ethmoid cells to the frontal process of the maxilla is called ANC [18]. This cell is in a close relationship with the lacrimal bone and affects the shape and size of the frontal recess (FR) anteriorly (**Figure 1**) [16]. Coronal CT images provide the clear identification of the ANC; however, sagittal views demonstrate the relation between the frontal sinus ostium, FR and ANC (**Figure 2**) [19]. The reported prevalence of ANC ranges from 15 to 92% [17, 19–22]. Also, Scribano et al. [23] reported that ANC was seen in nearly all patients. If there is an extensive pneumatization, it is thought that an enlarged ANC may narrow the drainage pathway of the frontal sinus and result in a chronic sinusitis [19]. However, no significant relationship was found between the ANC and frontal sinusitis [17, 20, 21].

http://dx.doi.org/10.5772/intechopen.69090

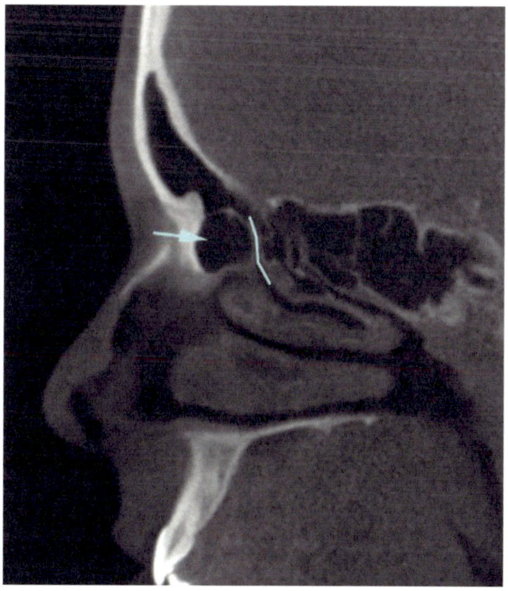

Figure 1. Sagittal CBCT images showing the large ANC (arrow) and its relation with the FR (line).

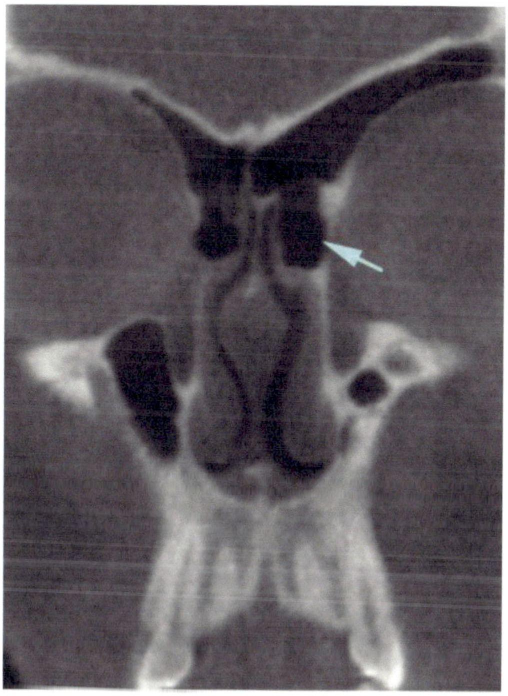

Figure 2. Coronal CBCT showing large ANC (arrow) on the left side which narrows the FR.

3.2. Infraorbital ethmoid cell (Haller's cell)

Haller's cells are defined as extramural migration of the posterior ethmoid cells situated beneath the floor of the orbit (the roof of the maxillary sinus), below the ethmoid bulla, most inferior portion of the lamina papyracea, and lateral to the uncinate process [18, 24]. The frequency rates of Haller's cell have been variously reported to be between 6 and 51% [17, 19–22, 24–27]. These cells are closely related with the maxillary sinus ostium, and according to its size, they may negatively affect the maxillary sinus ventilation (**Figure 3**). Although the presence of this anatomic variant was thought to be a predisposing factor for sinusitis, no statistically significant correlation was found in many studies [17, 20–22, 27]. However, Stackpole and Edelstein [26] classified Haller's cell as small, medium and large, and they found a statistically significant increase in maxillary sinus mucosal disease in patients with medium and large cells than the small ones.

3.3. Onodi (sphenoethmoid) cell

Extension of the most posterior ethmoid cells into the sphenoid sinus is termed as the onodi cell. This cell is located in the superolateral wall of the sphenoid sinus and is closely associated with the optic nerve (**Figure 4**) [18]. The reported prevalence of onodi cells is highly variable in the studies. The importance of these cells comes from risk of injury to the optic nerve when performing the sphenoid sinus surgery or the transsphenoidal approach to the hypophyseal fossa and a potential cause of incomplete sphenoidectomy [28]. The mean minimum of bone thickness between the onodi cell and optic nerve was reported as 0.08 mm by Thanaviratananich et al. [29] in a cadaveric study. Therefore, these nerves are particularly

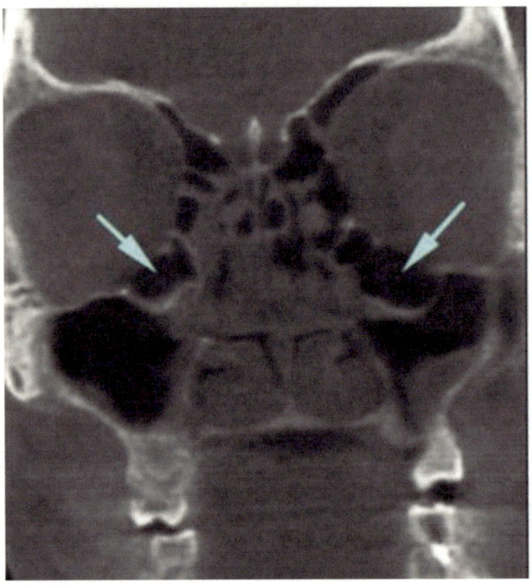

Figure 3. Bilateral huge infraorbital ethmoid cells.

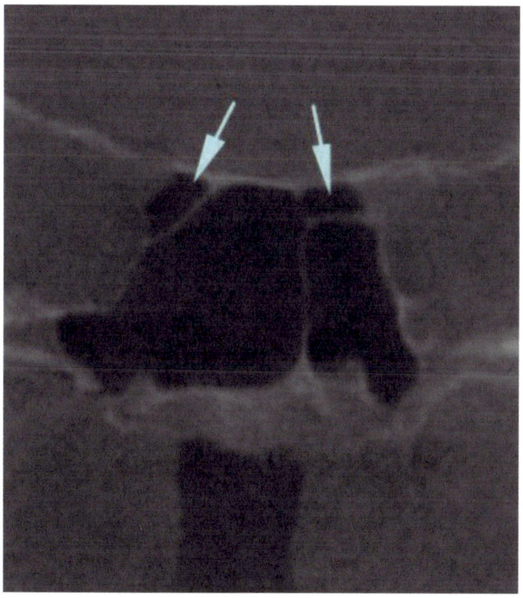

Figure 4. Coronal CBCT images. Bilateral onodi cell and its close relation with the optic nerve.

vulnerable to injury, and orbital complications such as blindness may occur during the surgery. Although optic nerve injury is the most important surgical complication in patients with onodi cells, there are other risks to vision as well. During the transsphenoidal surgery, onodi cells may limit the exposure of the sellar floor and should be removed [30, 31].

Onodi cells are not the single factor of the sphenoid sinusitis; however, with other predisposing factors, they may increase the prevalence of the sphenoiditis [32]. On the other hand, isolated mucoceles in an onodi cell may comprise the optic nerve and cause optic neuropathy [33, 34].

3.4. Concha bullosa

Intramural migration of the posterior ethmoid cells to the middle turbinate is called concha bullosa (CB) [18]. This anatomic variation was divided into three groups according to extent of the pneumatization: lamellar type (pneumatization in the lamellar portion), bulbous type (pneumatization in the bulbous portion; **Figure 5**), and extensive type (pneumatization in the both vertical lamellar and inferior bulbous portion) [35]. The prevalence of the CB varies from 4.6 to 89.5% [17, 20–22, 36–39]. This may be due to the different definition criteria for CB. While some researchers defined the CB as any degree of pneumatization in the middle concha regardless of location, the others restricted CB to specific locations.

CB is often associated with contralateral deviation of the nasal septum [16, 37]. It is still debated in the literature whether CB has a role in sinusitis aetiology. However, in most of the studies, no statistical significant relationship is found between the CB and maxillary sinusitis [17, 20–22, 36–39].

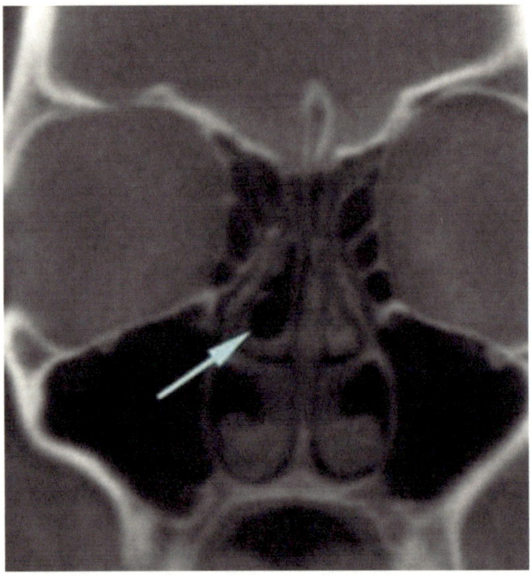

Figure 5. A bulbous type of the CB.

Pneumatization of the superior and inferior turbinate is also called superior and inferior concha bullosa. Superior and inferior CB are rare anatomic variations. If the pneumatization is extensive in the superior concha, it may cause headache with nasal obstruction and mucosal contact without any inflammation [19].

3.5. Uncinate bulla

Pneumatization of the uncinate process is referred to as uncinate bulla (UB) (**Figure 6**). This anatomic variation is believed to be extension of the ANC into the anterosuperior portion of the uncinate process [18]. UB may cause functional blockage of the osteomeatal unit. If the uncinate process is medially displaced and comes in contact with the middle turbinate, it may cause obstruction in OMU [19, 27, 39].

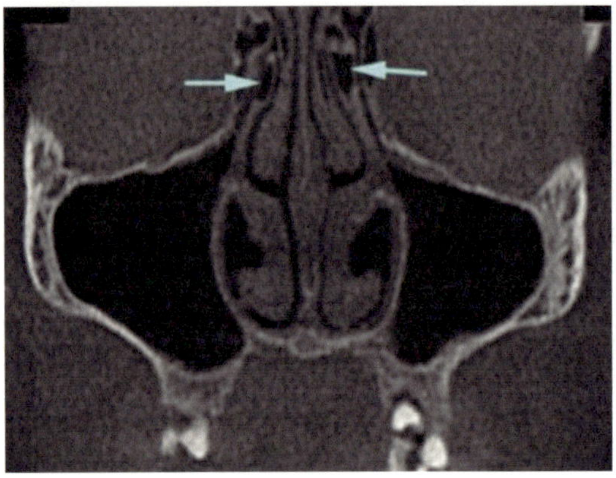

Figure 6. Bilateral uncinate process pneumatization.

3.6. Secondary concha

Secondary inferior, middle, or superior turbinate (**Figure 7**) are very rare anatomical variations. Embryologically, extra turbinates are consisted of secondary invagination and evaginations from the lateral nasal wall [40]. The incidence of the secondary middle turbinate is reported to be between the 2 and 14.3% [17, 19, 40, 41]. Secondary middle turbinate originates from the lateral nasal wall, and posterior part of the middle meatus and lamina papyracea may be damaged during the surgical operation for it [41].

3.7. Ethmomaxillary sinus

Extension of an enlarged posterior ethmoid cell above the maxillary sinus is called ethmomaxillary sinus (EMS). It is important to differentiate the maxillary sinus with septa and EMS [42–44]. While septate maxillary sinus drains into the middle meatus, EMS drains into the superior meatus (**Figure 8**) [43]. EMS is a rare anatomic variation, and the reported incidence of this anatomic variation ranges from 0.7 to 2% [42–44].

3.8. Sphenomaxillary plate

The partition between the ethmoid and maxillary sinus is called ethmomaxillary plate which is triangular in shape. In case of extensive pneumatization as a continuation of the ethmomaxillary plate, a thin-walled separating partition between the sphenoid and maxillary sinus is called sphenomaxillary plate (SMP) (**Figure 9**) [25, 45, 46]. It is important to identify this anatomic variation which may be mistaken for posterior ethmoid cells during transantral ethmoidectomy and increases the risk of inadvertent entry to the sphenoid sinus [45]. Reported incidence of the SMP was 11 [45], 14 [46], and 15% [19].

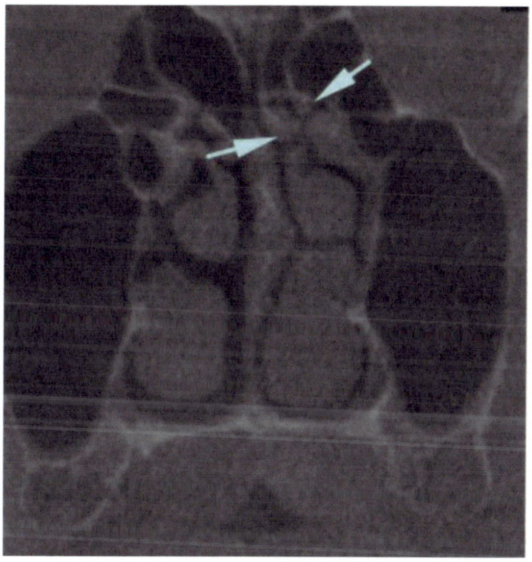

Figure 7. Coronal CBCT images showing the bifid superior turbinate.

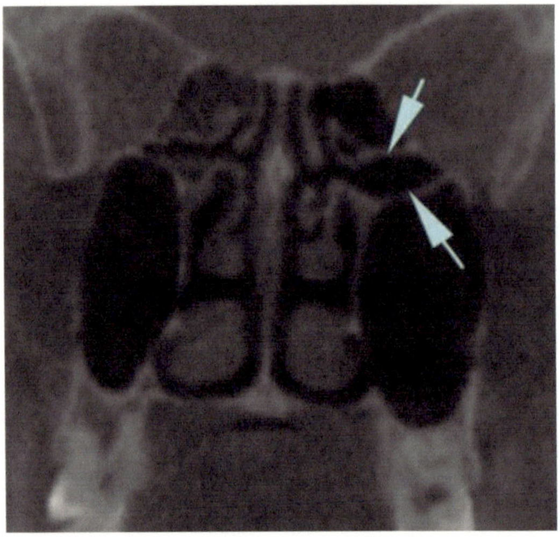

Figure 8. Left-side ethmomaxillary sinus and its drainage into the superior meatus.

3.9. Sphenoid sinus ICA and MN relations

Sphenoid sinus is located within the body of the sphenoid bone and closely related with the numerous neurovascular structures. ICA and MN lie adjacent to the lateral wall of the sphenoid sinus and during their passage may produce variable bulging into the sinus [18]. These neurovascular structures are covered by a thin bone separating the ICA and MN from the sphenoid sinus mucosa. Sometimes, this bony canal covering is found to be partially dehiscent, and ICA and MN are only covered by the mucoperiosteum. In this situation, neurovascular structures become vulnerable to infection and damage [15, 47].

The prevalence of the ICA bulging (**Figure 10**) into the sphenoid sinus varies from 3 to 41% [15, 47–51]. In case of bulging, an ICA injury may occur due to a trauma or a complication of sinus disease. If the surgeon is not aware of this variation, fatal haemorrhage can occur; it is

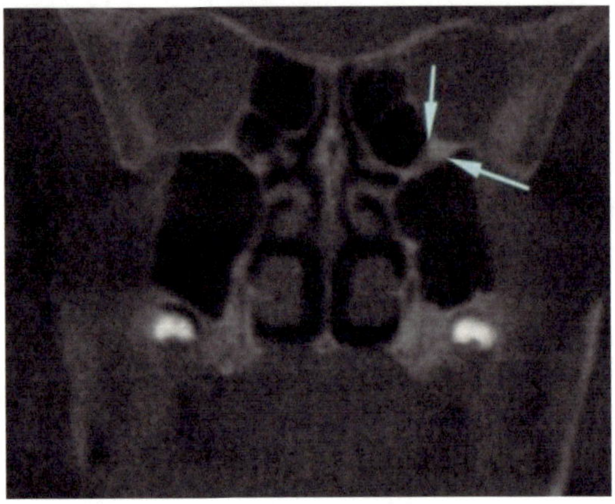

Figure 9. Left-side SMP.

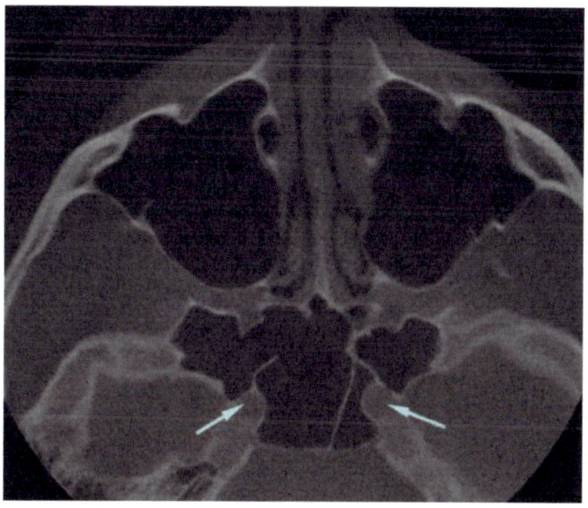

Figure 10. ICA protrusion into the sphenoid sinus bilaterally.

hardly possible to control the bleeding from this artery, and neurological sequelae are inevitable [15, 51]. Another complication during the surgery is if the septum in the sphenoid sinus (**Figure 11**) adheres to the wall of the ICA, the surgeon must be careful about not fracturing it to avoid the artery damage [18, 50].

The frequency rates of MN bulging (**Figure 12**) have been reported to be between 14.2 and 30.3% [47, 50, 51]. MN is also at risk during sphenoid sinus surgery, and sinus pathology may be related with the trigeminal neuralgia [52].

3.10. Pneumatization of the pterygoid, anterior versus posterior clinoid process

There are two definitions about the pterygoid process (PP) pneumatization (**Figure 13**) in the literature. If there is an extensive sphenoid sinus pneumatization that extends beyond a horizontal plane crossing the VC [51], or a plane between the VC and FR [15, 47], it is considered

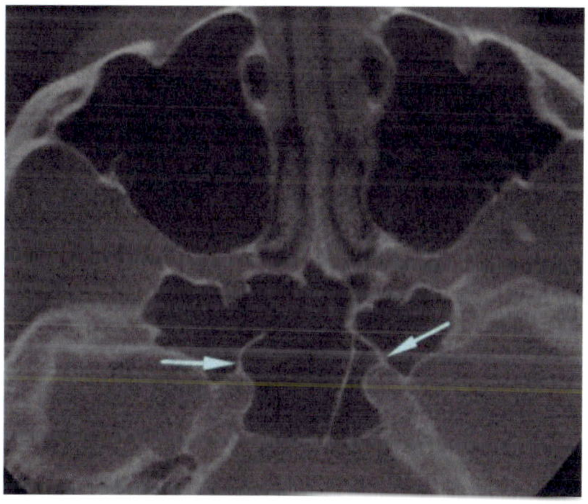

Figure 11. Axial CBCT images. Sphenoid sinus septum adheres to the ICA wall bilaterally.

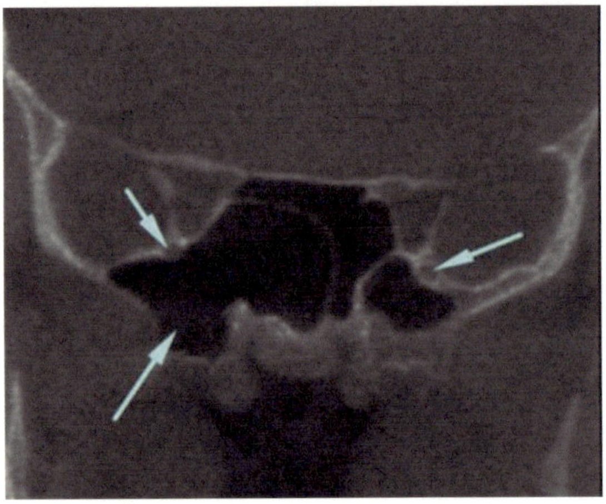

Figure 12. Bilateral MN protrusion into the sphenoid sinus.

that patient has PP pneumatization. If the sinus expands to the pterygoid processes, the sinus floor creates a definite ridge where the vidian channel is located. PP pneumatization may lead to the formation of a potential cavity for the accumulation of sinus-associated purulent exudate [47]. PP pneumatization is a very important surgical route for access to the middle part of the skull base without brain retraction. This route can be used in the endoscopic repair of the leak of cerebrospinal fluid and endoscopic biopsy of skull-base lesions [53].

Pneumatization of the sphenoid sinus may extend into the anterior (**Figure 14**) or posterior clinoid (**Figure 15**) process. In most of the study, ACP pneumatization was found to be significantly associated with the optic nerve protrusion [15, 47, 48, 51].

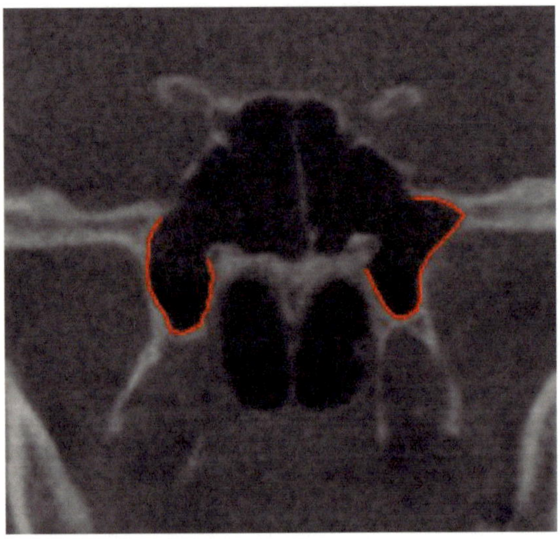

Figure 13. Coronal CBCT images show the bilateral remarkable PP pneumatization.

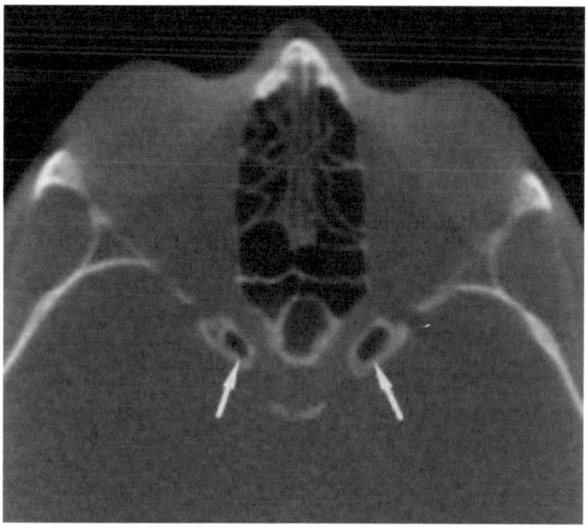

Figure 14. Extensive pneumatization of the sphenoid sinus to the bilateral ACP.

The posterior clinoid process pneumatization prevalence is reported to be 1% by Lu et al. [54].

3.11. Nasal septum deviation and pneumatization

Congenital or acquired deviation could be seen in the nasal septum (**Figure 16**). Deviated nasal septum may compress the middle turbinate laterally and narrow the middle meatus [52]. The reported prevalence of nasal septum deviation ranges from 18 to 75.9% [20, 21, 25, 27, 29, 55].

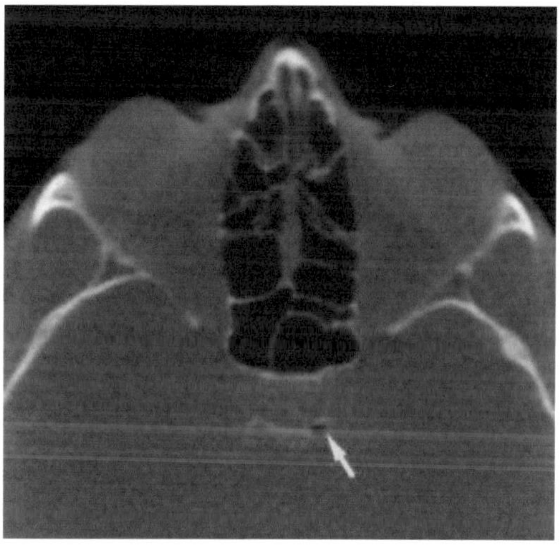

Figure 15. Posterior clinoid process pneumatization on the left side.

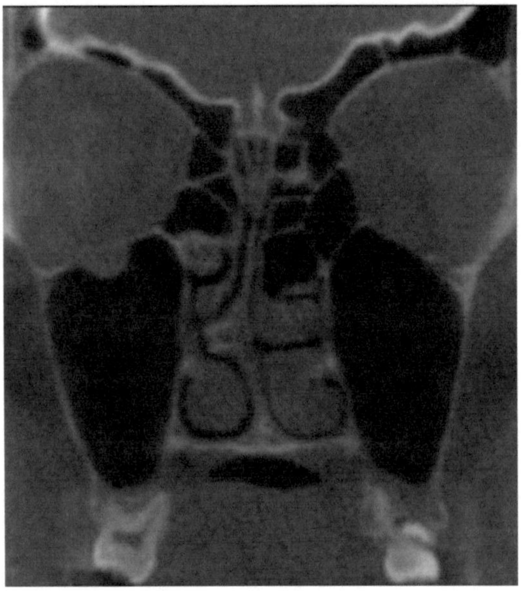

Figure 16. Nasal septum deviation to the right side with a septal spur.

Air cells are usually located within the posterosuperior portion of the nasal septum (**Figure 17**) and related with the sphenoid sinus. These cells may also be affected by any inflammation within the paranasal sinus [18]. This anatomic variation is generally not important but sometimes may narrow the sphenoethmoid recess [52].

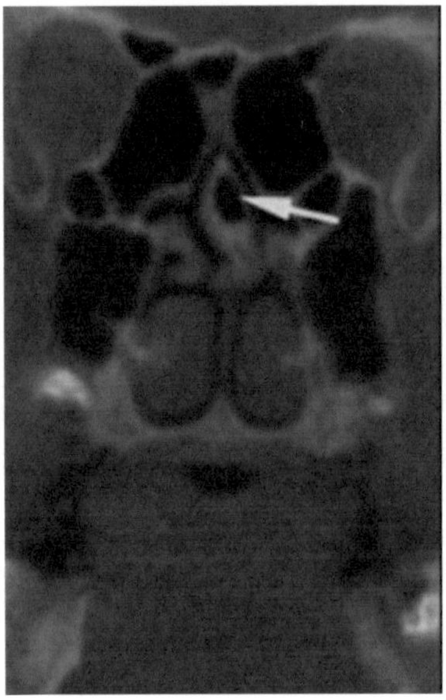

Figure 17. Nasal septum pneumatization.

3.12. Interfrontal sinus septa cell

Interfrontal sinus septa cells (IFSSCs) are defined as discrete air cells in the frontal sinus septum (**Figure 18**) [56]. These cells drain into the one of the FR and are well defined in the coronal and axial scans [57]. The incidence rate in the literature is reported as 12.4 [56] and 14% [58].

3.13. Supraorbital ethmoid cell

Supraorbital ethmoid cell (SOEC) is formed by anterior ethmoid cells that pneumatize the roof of the orbit behind the posterior wall of the frontal sinus (**Figure 19**) [25]. If the pathology in these cells cannot be determined, it may lead to failure of operations performed on the frontal sinus. On coronal images, the presence of bony septum between the ethmoid complex and the recess separates the frontal sinus from the SOEC [18]. These cells drain into the lateral aspect of the FR [57]. Because of the close relation between the SOEC and anterior ethmoidal artery, enlarging the SOEC could risk damage to the artery [59].

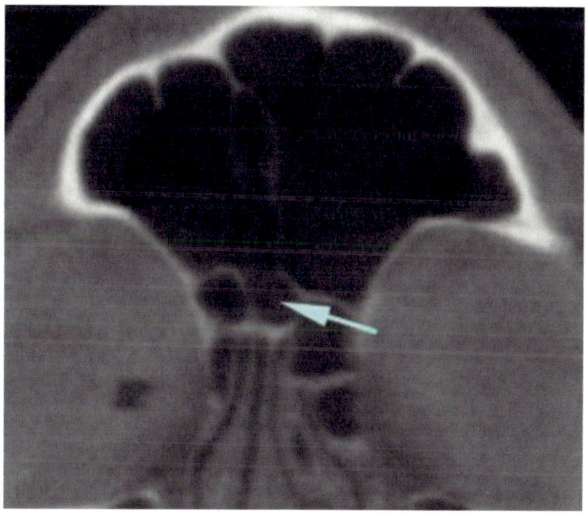

Figure 18. The coronal image shows the IFSSC.

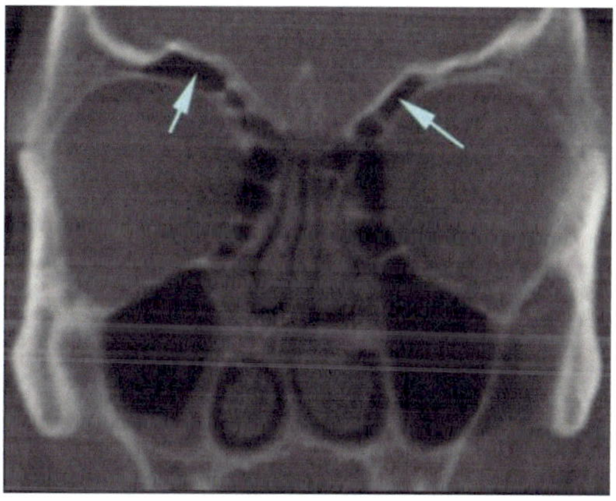

Figure 19. Bilateral supraorbital ethmoid cells.

3.14. Crista galli pneumatization

The pneumatized crista galli (**Figure 20**) is associated with the frontal recess, and with the obstruction of this ostium, chronic sinusitis or mucocele formation may occur in crista galli [18].

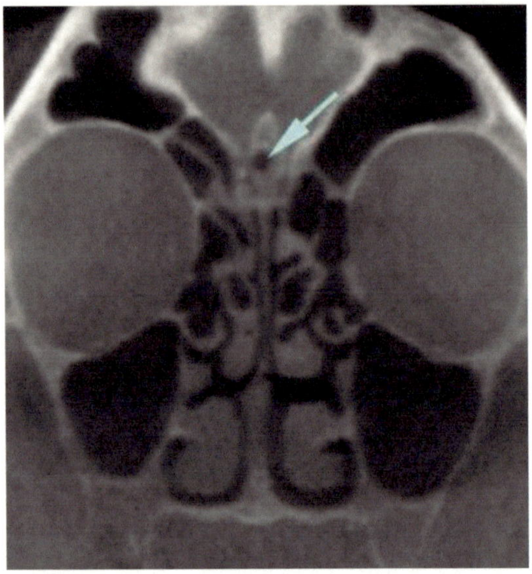

Figure 20. Aeration of the crista galli.

4. Conclusion

Paranasal sinus variations are very common. Before the sinus surgery, CBCT is the best imaging method with lower radiation dose for the determination of sinonasal anatomy.

Author details

Kaan Orhan[1*], Secil Aksoy[2] and Ulas Oz[3]

*Address all correspondence to: call53@yahoo.com

1 Faculty of Dentistry, Department of Dentomaxillofacial Radiology, Ankara University, Ankara, Turkey

2 Faculty of Dentistry, Department of Dentomaxillofacial Radiology, Near East University, Nicosia, Northern Cyprus

3 Faculty of Dentistry, Department of Orthodontics, Near East University, Nicosia, Northern Cyprus

References

[1] Keir J. Why do we have paranasal sinuses?. The Journal of Laryngology & Otology. 2009;**123**(1):4–8

[2] Gallup AC, Hack GD. Human paranasal sinuses and selective brain cooling: A ventilation system activated by yawning? Medical Hypotheses. 2011;**77**(6):970–973

[3] Koertvelyessy T. Relationships between the frontal sinus and climatic conditions: A skeletal approach to cold adaptation. American Journal of Physical Anthropology. 1972;**37**(2):161–172

[4] Irmak MK, Korkmaz A, Erogul O. Selective brain cooling seems to be a mechanism leading to human craniofacial diversity observed in different geographical regions. Medical Hypotheses. 2004;**63**(6):974–979

[5] Ebrahimnejad H, Zarch SH, Langaroodi AJ. Diagnostic efficacy of digital waters' and Caldwell's radiographic views for evaluation of sinonasal area. Journal of Dentistry (Tehran). 2016;**13**(5):357–364

[6] Aygun N, Zinreich SJ. Radiology of the nasal cavity and paranasal sinuses. In: Cummings Otolaryngology: Head & Neck Surgery. 5th ed. Philadelphia, PA: Elsevier Mosby. 2010 pg: 662–663

[7] Konen E, Faibel M, Kleinbaum Y, Wolf M, Lusky A, Hoffman C, Eyal A, Tadmor R. The value of the occipitomental (Waters') view in diagnosis of sinusitis: A comparative study with computed tomography. Clinical Radiology. 2000;**55**(11):856–860

[8] Fatterpekar GM, Delman BN, Som PM. Imaging the paranasal sinuses: Where we are and where we are going. The Anatomical Record. 2008;**291**(11):1564–1572

[9] Scarfe WC, Farman AG, Sukovic P. Clinical applications of cone-beam computed tomography in dental practice. Journal-Canadian Dental Association. 2006;**72**(1):75

[10] Phothikhun S, Suphanantachat S, Chuenchompoonut V, Nisapakultorn K. Cone-beam computed tomographic evidence of the association between periodontal bone loss and mucosal thickening of the maxillary sinus. Journal of Periodontology. 2012;**83**(5):557–564

[11] Altschuler MD, Censor Y, Eggermont PP, Herman GT, Kuo YH, Lewitt RM, McKay M, Tuy HK, Udupa JK, Yau MM. Demonstration of a software package for the reconstruction of the dynamically changing structure of the human heart from cone beam x-ray projections. Journal of Medical Systems. 1980;**4**(2):289–304

[12] Brüllmann DD, Schmidtmann I, Hornstein S, Schulze RK. Correlation of cone beam computed tomography (CBCT) findings in the maxillary sinus with dental diagnoses: A retrospective cross-sectional study. Clinical Oral Investigations. 2012;**16**(4):1023–1029

[13] Márquez S, Tessema B, Clement PA, Schaefer SD. Development of the ethmoid sinus and extramural migration: The anatomical basis of this paranasal sinus. The Anatomical Record. 2008;**291**(11):1535–1553

[14] Dasar U, Gokce E. Evaluation of variations in sinonasal region with computed tomography. World Journal of Radiology. 2016;**8**(1):98

[15] Sirikci A, Bayazıt YA, Bayram M, Mumbuc S, Güngör K, Kanlıkama M. Variations of sphenoid and related structures. European Radiology. 2000;**10**(5):844–848

[16] Maroldi R, Borghesi A, Maculotti P. CT and MR anatomy of paranasal sinuses: Key elements. In: Imaging in Treatment Planning for Sinonasal Diseases. Berlin, Heidelberg: Springer; 2005. pp. 9–27

[17] Sivaslı E, Sirikçi A, Bayazýt Y, Gümüsburun E, Erbagci H, Bayram M, Kanlýkama M. Anatomic variations of the paranasal sinus area in pediatric patients with chronic sinusitis. Surgical and Radiologic Anatomy. 2002;**24**(6):399–404

[18] Som PM, Curtin HD. Head and Neck Imaging. 5th ed. St. Louis, MO. Elsevier Mosby. 2011 pg: 120–124

[19] Kantarci M, Karasen RM, Alper F, Onbas O, Okur A, Karaman A. Remarkable anatomic variations in paranasal sinus region and their clinical importance. European Journal of Radiology. 2004;**50**(3):296–302

[20] Al-Qudah M. The relationship between anatomical variations of the sino-nasal region and chronic sinusitis extension in children. International Journal of Pediatric Otorhinolaryngology. 2008;**72**(6):817–821

[21] Jun Kim H, Jung Cho M, Lee JW, Tae Kim Y, Kahng H, Sung Kim H, Hahm KH. The relationship between anatomic variations of paranasal sinuses and chronic sinusitis in children. Acta Oto-Laryngologica. 2006;**126**(10):1067–1072

[22] Nitinavakarn B, Thanaviratananich S, Sangsilp N. Anatomical variations of the lateral nasal wall and paranasal sinuses: A CT study for endoscopic sinus surgery (ESS) in Thai patients. Journal of the Medical Association of Thailand. 2005;**88**(6):763–768

[23] Scribano E, Ascenti G, Cascio F, Racchiusa S, Salamone I. Computerized tomography in the evaluation of anatomic variations of the ostiomeatal complex. La Radiologia Medica. 1993;**86**(3):195–199

[24] Bašić N, Bašić V, Jukić T, Bašić M, Jelić M, Hat J. Computed tomographic imaging to determine the frequency of anatomical variations in pneumatization of the ethmoid bone. European Archives of Oto-Rhino-Laryngology. 1999;**256**(2):69–71

[25] Arslan H, Aydınlıoğlu A, Bozkurt M, Egeli E. Anatomic variations of the paranasal sinuses: CT examination for endoscopic sinus surgery. Auris Nasus Larynx. 1999;**26**(1): 39–48

[26] Stackpole SA, Edelstein DR. The anatomic relevance of the Haller cell in sinusitis. American Journal of Rhinology. 1997;**11**(3):219–223

[27] Azila A, Irfan M, Rohaizan Y, Shamim AK. The prevalence of anatomical variations in osteomeatal unit in patients with chronic rhinosinusitis. The Medical Journal of Malaysia. 2011;**66**(3):191–194

[28] Hwang SH, Joo YH, Seo JH, Cho JH, Kang JM. Analysis of sphenoid sinus in the operative plane of endoscopic transsphenoidal surgery using computed tomography. European Archives of Oto-Rhino-Laryngology. 2014;**271**(8):2219–2225

[29] Thanaviratananich S, Chaisiwamongkol K, Kraitrakul S, Tangsawad W. The prevalence of an Onodi cell in adult Thai cadavers. Ear, Nose & Throat Journal. 2003;**82**(3):200

[30] İmre A, Pinar E, Yüceer N, Songu M, Olgun Y, Aladağ İ. Does Onodi cell limit the exposure of sella during transsphenoidal pituitary surgery? Kulak Burun Bogaz Ihtisas Dergisi: KBB=Journal of Ear, Nose, and Throat. 2014;**25**(2):82–86

[31] Shin JH, Kim SW, Hong YK, Jeun SS, Kang SG, Kim SW, Cho JH, Park YJ. The Onodi cell: An obstacle to sellar lesions with a transsphenoidal approach. Otolaryngology—Head and Neck Surgery. 2011;**145**(6):1040–1042

[32] Senturk M, Guler I, Azgin I, Sakarya EU, Ovet G, Alatas N, Tolu I, Erdur O. The role of Onodi cells in sphenoiditis: results of multiplanar reconstruction of computed tomography scanning. Brazilian journal of otorhinolaryngology. 2017;83:88–93

[33] Kitagawa K, Hayasaka S, Shimizu K, Nagaki Y. Optic neuropathy produced by a compressed mucocele in an Onodi cell. American Journal of Ophthalmology. 2003;**135**(2):253–254

[34] Lim CT, Dillon WP, McDermott MW. Mucocele involving the anterior clinoid process: MR and CT findings. American Journal of Neuroradiology. 1999;**20**(2):287–290

[35] Bolger WE, Parsons DS, Butzin CA. Paranasal sinus bony anatomic variations and mucosal abnormalities: CT analysis for endoscopic sinus surgery. The Laryngoscope. 1991;**101**(1):56–64

[36] Haruna S, Sawada K, Nakajima T, Moriyama H. Relationship between pediatric sinusitis and middle turbinate pneumatization—ethmoidal sinus pyocele thought to be caused by middle turbinate pneumatization. International Journal of Pediatric Otorhinolaryngology. 2005;**69**(3):375–379

[37] Stallman JS, Lobo JN, Som PM. The incidence of concha bullosa and its relationship to nasal septal deviation and paranasal sinus disease. American Journal of Neuroradiology. 2004;**25**(9):1613–1618

[38] Smith KD, Edwards PC, Saini TS, Norton NS. The prevalence of concha bullosa and nasal septal deviation and their relationship to maxillary sinusitis by volumetric tomography. International Journal of Dentistry. 2010;**2010**

[39] Hatipoglu HG, Cetin MA, Yüksel E. Concha bullosa types: Their relationship with sinusitis, ostiomeatal and frontal recess disease. Diagnostic and Interventional Radiology. 2005;**11**(3):145

[40] El-Shazly AE, Poirrier AL, Cabay J, Lefebvre PP. Anatomical variations of the lateral nasal wall: The secondary and accessory middle turbinates. Clinical Anatomy. 2012;**25**(3):340–346

[41] Ozcan KM, Selcuk A, Özcan I, Akdogan O, Dere H. Anatomical variations of nasal turbinates. Journal of Craniofacial Surgery. 2008;**19**(6):1678–1682

[42] Ozcan KM, Selcuk A, Oruk V, Sarikaya Y, Dere H. Ethmomaxillary sinus. European Archives of Oto-Rhino-Laryngology. 2008;**265**(2):185–188

[43] Sirikçi A, Bayazıt YA, Bayram M, Kanlıkama M. Ethmomaxillary sinus: A particular anatomic variation of the paranasal sinuses. European Radiology. 2004;**14**(2):281–285

[44] Selcuk A, Ozcan KM, Akdogan O, Bilal N, Dere H. Variations of maxillary sinus and accompanying anatomical and pathological structures. Journal of Craniofacial Surgery. 2008;**19**(1):159–164

[45] Nouraei SA, Elisay AR, Dimarco A, Abdi R, Majidi H, Madani SA, Andrews PJ. Variations in paranasal sinus anatomy: Implications for the pathophysiology of chronic rhinosinusitis and safety of endoscopic sinus surgery. Journal of Otolaryngology—Head and Neck Surgery. 2009;**38**(1):32

[46] Meloni F, Mini R, Rovasio S, Stomeo F, Teatini GP. Anatomic variations of surgical importance in ethmoid labyrinth and sphenoid sinus. A study of radiological anatomy. Surgical and Radiologic Anatomy. 1992;**14**(1):65–70

[47] Kazkayasi M, Karadeniz Y, Arikan OK. Anatomic variations of the sphenoid sinus on computed tomography. Rhinology. 2005;**43**(2):109–114

[48] Basak S, Karaman CZ, Akdilli A, Mutlu C, Odabası O, Erpek G. Evaluation of some important anatomical variations and dangerous areas of the paranasal sinuses by CT for safer endonasal surgery. Rhinology. 1998;**36**:162–167

[49] Güldner C, Pistorius SM, Diogo I, Bien S, Sesterhenn A, Werner JA. Analysis of pneumatization and neurovascular structures of the sphenoid sinus using cone-beam tomography (CBT). Acta Radiologica. 2012;**53**(2):214–219

[50] Unal B, Bademci G, Bilgili YK, Batay F, Avci E. Risky anatomic variations of sphenoid sinus for surgery. Surgical and Radiologic Anatomy. 2006;**28**(2):195–201

[51] Hewaidi GH, Omami GM. Anatomic variation of sphenoid sinus and related structures in Libyan population: CT scan study. Libyan Journal of Medicine. 2008;**3**(3):1–9

[52] Beale TJ, Madani G, Morley SJ. Imaging of the paranasal sinuses and nasal cavity: Normal anatomy and clinically relevant anatomical variants. Seminars in Ultrasound, CT and MRI. 2009;**30**(1):2–16

[53] Wang J, Bidari S, Inoue K, Yang H, Rhoton A Jr. Extensions of the sphenoid sinus: A new classification. Neurosurgery. 2010;**66**(4):797–816

[54] Lu Y, Pan J, Qi S, Shi J, Zhang XA, Wu K. Pneumatization of the sphenoid sinus in Chinese: The differences from Caucasian and its application in the extended transsphenoidal approach. Journal of Anatomy. 2011;**219**(2):132–142

[55] Aktas D, Kalcioglu MT, Kutlu R, Ozturan O, Oncel S. The relationship between the concha bullosa, nasal septal deviation and sinusitis. Rhinology. 2003;**41**(2):103–106

[56] Meyer TK, Kocak M, Smith MM, Smith TL. Coronal computed tomography analysis of frontal cells. American Journal of Rhinology. 2003;**17**(3):163–168

[57] Cho JH, Citardi MJ, Lee WT, Sautter NB, Lee HM, Yoon JH, Hong SC, Kim JK. Comparison of frontal pneumatization patterns between Koreans and Caucasians. Otolaryngology—Head and Neck Surgery. 2006;**135**(5):780–786

[58] Lee WT, Kuhn FA, Citardi MJ. 3D computed tomographic analysis of frontal recess anatomy in patients without frontal sinusitis. Otolaryngology—Head and Neck Surgery. 2004;**131**(3):164–173

[59] Zhang L, Han D, Ge W, Tao J, Wang X, Li Y, Zhou B. Computed tomographic and endoscopic analysis of supraorbital ethmoid cells. Otolaryngology—Head and Neck Surgery. 2007;**137**(4):562–568

Section 4

Nasal Spacers

Chapter 4

Nasal Packing after Functional Endoscopic Sinus Surgery

Tang-Chuan Wang and Hung-Ta Hsiao

Additional information is available at the end of the chapter

http://dx.doi.org/10.5772/intechopen.68993

Abstract

This chapter was to have a systematic review and meta-analysis on the available literature in order to compare the efficacy and postoperative outcomes of nasal packing (absorbable vs. nonabsorbable) after treatment of chronic rhinosinusitis with functional endoscopic sinus surgery (FESS). The systematic review included five studies with 241 nasal cavities in each treatment group. The prevalence of synechia in the absorbable groups ranged from 4.6 to 8.0% while nonabsorbable groups ranged from 8.0 to 35.7%. The absorbable group had a lower postoperative bleeding; however, there were no clear findings on postoperative pain. Postoperative edema was in general similar among groups, and no consistent findings were found on bleeding and pain while removing packing. The meta-analysis included two studies using the same type of packing material. The combined OR (0.33, 95% CI = 0.04–2.78) for postoperative synechia did not significantly favor (P = 0.016308) absorbable packing over nonabsorbable packing. The available literature showed that there is some evidence that absorbable nasal packing may provide superior outcomes to nonabsorbable packing after FESS. However, lack of homogeneity between these studies makes it impossible to have a definitive conclusion.

Keywords: absorbable, bleeding, efficacy, epistaxis, FESS, functional endoscopic sinus surgery, meta-analysis, nasal, nonabsorbable, packing, synechia

1. Introduction

Chronic rhinosinusitis is an extremely common condition affecting millions of individuals worldwide. Up to approximately 16% of the adult population in the United States were reported to have suffered from it [1, 2]. Chronic rhinosinusitis can have a significant negative impact on quality of life [3], and therefore, treatment is usually required. Although chronic rhinosinusitis can usually be managed pharmacologically, some patients do not respond well and require surgery [2].

The most commonly used surgical approach for the management of chronic rhinosinusitis perhaps is functional endoscopic sinus surgery (FESS) [4, 5]. It aims to improve or restore drainage and airflow on affected sinuses [2]. FESS is effective in more than 90% of patients [6] and significantly improves quality of life [7]; nonetheless, postoperative complications such as bleeding and adhesions (synechia) are quite common [8]. Due to this reason, after FESS, the nasal cavity is often packed with material designed to stop bleeding, reduce clot formation, lower the risk of synechia, and promote healing [8, 9]. Nonabsorbable nasal packing was applied after FESS traditionally [7]; nonetheless, patients seem not be able to tolerate the packing and its removal [10]. Absorbable nasal packing was introduced more recently and appears to be well tolerated by patients [11, 12].

There were a number of studies comparing the efficacy of nonabsorbable and absorbable nasal packing after FESS [8–14]; however, the results on if a method is better than another or if the methods used had a comparable efficacy were conflicting among the studies. In an effort to gain a better understanding of the efficacy and other outcomes on nonabsorbable vs. absorbable nasal packing after FESS for the treatment of chronic rhinosinusitis, we have conducted a systematic review and a meta-analysis of the available literature. Among the literature, we only include randomized trials and examined postoperative synechia as the key indicator of nasal packing efficacy in our meta-analysis.

2. Material and methods

2.1. Searching strategy

Combinations of the following search terms, FESS, rhinosinusitis, bleeding, gelatin, hyaluronic acid, carboxymethylated cellulose, CMC, and packing, were used on Medline, Current Contents, and the Cochrane databases on January 31, 2013.

2.2. Studies selection

Studies meet following criteria were considered for inclusion in this systematic review and meta-analysis—Studies published in English, randomized clinical trials, reported on postoperative pain, edema, synechia/adhesion and/or bleeding/hemostasis. Studies were excluded if they did not meet those criteria.

2.3. Extraction of data

Two independent reviewers were employed to extract data. If there were any disagreements, a third reviewer would be consulted. The following data were extracted for each eligible study: authors, year of publication, number of nasal cavities packed per treatment group, age of participants, sex distribution of participants, the type of nasal packing used, postoperative treatment, the time to removal of packing, the incidence of postoperative synechia, the incidence of postoperative bleeding, postoperative pain, postoperative edema, and bleeding and pain on removal of packing.

The incidence of postoperative synechia for absorbable nasal packing vs. nonabsorbable nasal packing was the primary outcome for our meta-analysis.

2.4. Analysis of data

Binary outcomes and comparisons made for absorbable nasal packing vs. nonabsorbable nasal packing were calculated from odds ratios (ORs) with 95% confidence intervals (CIs). A χ^2-based test of homogeneity was implemented, and the inconsistency index (I2) statistic was determined. If I2 was >50%, the studies were considered to be heterogeneous; if I2 was >75%, the studies were considered to be highly heterogeneous; and if I2 was <25%, the studies were considered to be homogeneous. If the I2 statistic (>50%) indicated heterogeneity existed between studies, a random-effects model was calculated; otherwise, a fixed-effects model was calculated. Pooled summary statistics for ORs of the individual studies are reported, a P value < 0.05 was taken to indicate statistical significance. All analyses were performed using Comprehensive Meta-Analysis statistical software, version 2.0 (Biostat, Englewood, NJ).

3. Results

3.1. Search of literature

Of total of 124 records that were retrieved from the database search, 106 were excluded after title/abstract review, 13 were excluded after full-text review, and five were included in the systematic review with two of these five studies also included in the meta-analysis of postoperative synechia.

3.2. Characteristics of study

Table 1 summarized the systematic review, which included the studies characteristics [8, 11–13, 15]. A total of 241 nasal cavities were treated in each group for all studies combined and the number of nasal cavities treated in each study ranged from 30 to 100. Four of the five studies [8, 11, 13, 15] reported the age of study participants which ranging from 35.7 to 43.2 years among three studies [8, 13, 15] and 54.0 years in one study [11]. The same four studies [8, 11, 13, 15] also reported the sex distribution of the participants, with the ratio of males ranging from 54 to 67%. For the absorbable nasal packing materials, MeroGel® was used in two studies [8, 12], while Cutanplast [15], carboxymethylated cellulose (CMC) foam [13], and NasoPore [11] were used in the other three studies, respectively. For nonabsorbable nasal packing material, Merocel was used in three studies [8, 11, 15], polyvinyl alcohol sponges [12], and routine nasal packing (cotton gauze placed in a latex glove finger) [13] were used in the remaining two studies respectively. Among the five studies, four [8, 12, 13, 15] of which reported on postoperative treatments with the administration of various antibiotics, three [8, 11, 13] of which reported on the time to packing removal which ranging from 1 to 7 days.

First author (year)	Nasal cavities packed Abs vs. Nonabs	Age (years)	Sex (male %)	Absorbable packing	Nonabsorbable packing	Postoperative treatment	Time to packing removal
Cho (2012)	100 vs. 100	35.7	64	Cutanplast	Merocel	2nd generation cephalosporin or clarithromycin, analgesics as needed, prednisone	NA
Miller (2003)	37 vs. 37	39.1	54%	MeroGel®	Merocel	Cefuroxime, saline nasal spray and nasal irrigation	Postoperative day 5–7
Berlucchi (2009)	44 vs. 44	NA	NA	MeroGel®	PVA sponge	Amoxicillin + clavulanic acid, non-aspirin analgesics as needed, saline nasal spray	NA
Szczygielski (2010)	30 vs. 30	43.2	62%	CMC foam	Routine packing[a]	Cefazolin sodium, decongestants	Postoperative day 1
Shoman (2009)	30 vs. 30	54	67	NasoPore	Merocel	NA	Postoperative day 7

[a]Cotton gauze placed in a latex glove finger.

Abs, absorbable nasal packing material; CMC, carboxymethylated cellulose; NA, data not available; Nonabs, nonabsorbable nasal packing material; PVA, polyvinyl alcohol.

Table 1. Characteristics of studies included in the systematic review.

3.3. Outcomes of study

Three studies [8, 12, 13] reported the prevalence of synechia and were ranged from 4.6 to 8.0% in the absorbable packing groups and from 8.0 to 35.7% in the nonabsorbable packing groups. The follow-up duration for monitoring of postoperative synechia was 12 weeks in one study [12] and 8 weeks in two studies [8, 13]. Two studies [11, 13] reported postoperative bleeding data and both found decreased bleeding in the absorbable group compared to the nonabsorbable group. The same two studies also reported postoperative pain data with one found that pain was less in the nonabsorbable group [11], while the other found the pain was considerable less in the absorbable group [13]. Postoperative edema results were reported on three studies [8, 11, 12]; one [12] of which found that edema was less pronounced in the absorbable group compared with the nonabsorbable group, while the other two [8, 11] found no clear differences in edema between groups. Two studies [11, 15] reported on bleeding and pain on packing removal, respectively. One study [11] found that pain and bleeding were similar among groups, while the other study [15] found that pain and bleeding were both markedly reduced in the absorbable group compared with the nonabsorbable group. See **Table 2** for the aforementioned assessments which the timing varied between studies.

	Abs vs. Nonabs					
First author (year)	**Synechia**	**Postoperative bleeding**	**Postoperative pain**	**Postoperative edema**	**Bleeding on packing removal**	**Pain on packing removal**
Cho (2012)	NA	NA	NA	NA	59 vs. 91%	1.01 ± 0.16 vs. 2.37 ± 0.19
Miller (2003)	8.0 vs. 8.0% (8 weeks)	NA	NA	0.70 ± 0.45 vs. 0.71 ± 0.45 (8 weeks)	NA	NA
Berlucchi (2009)	4.6 vs. 29.7% (12 weeks)	NA	NA	43.2 vs. 58.4%	NA	NA
Szczygielski (2010)	6.7 vs. 35.7% (8 weeks)	13.3 vs. 6.7%	5.5 (3-9) vs. 0.962 (0-4) (24 h)	NA	NA	NA
Shoman (2009)	NA	3.67 ± 2.45 vs. 3.44 ± 2.01 (1 st week)	3.33 ± 2.50 vs. 3.70 ± 2.98 (1 st week)	2.78 ± 2.52 vs. 2.78 ± 2.36 (1st week)	0.90 ± 0.55 vs. 0.83 ± 0.53	4.03 ± 2.80 vs. 3.97 ± 2.72

Abs, absorbable nasal packing material; Nonabs, nonabsorbable nasal packing material; NA, data not available; VAS, visual analogue scale.

Table 2. Summary of outcomes for studies included in the systematic review.

3.4. Assessment quality

Table 3 highlighted the quality of the studies included in the systematic review. Not all studies [8, 13] had comprehensive information, and several studies [8, 11, 12] did not have outcome assessor, care provider, and/or patient blinding. However, the studies generally had

First author (year)	Method of randomization used	Groups similar at baseline regarding the most important prognostic indicators	Eligibility criteria specified	Outcome assessor blinded	Care provider blinded	Patient blinded	Point estimates and measures of variability presented for the primary outcome measures	Analysis included an intention-to-treat analysis
Cho (2012)	Y	Y	Y	Y	Y	Y	Y	N
Miller (2003)	Y	NA	Y	Y	N	N	Y	Y
Berlucchi (2009)	Y	Y	Y	Y	N	N	Y	Y
Szczygielski (2010)	Y	NA	Y	NA	NA	NA	Y	Y
Shoman (2009)	Y	Y	Y	Y	N	Y	Y	Y

N, no; NA, information not available or not applicable; Y, yes.

Table 3. Quality assessment of studies included in the systematic review.

characteristics consistent with being high quality trials. The study reported by Cho et al. [15] met all of the quality criteria aside from not including an intention-to-treat analysis.

3.5. Postoperative synechia meta-analysis

Figure 1 summarized the results of the two studies [8, 12], which were included in the meta-analysis of postoperative synechia. A random-effects model of analysis was used because there was a significant heterogeneity between the two studies for this outcome (Q = 3.492, I2 = 71.37%, P = 0.062). The combined OR for postoperative synechia did not significantly favor absorbable nasal packing over nonabsorbable nasal packing or vice-versa (P = 0.308).

Authors	Odds ratio	Lower limit	Upper limit	Z Value	P Value	Odds ratio and 95% CI	Relative Weight
Miller et al 2003	1.00	0.19	5.29	0.00	1.000		49.06
Berlucchi et al 2009	0.11	0.02	0.54	-2.73	0.006		50.94
Combined	0.33	0.04	2.78	-1.02	0.308		

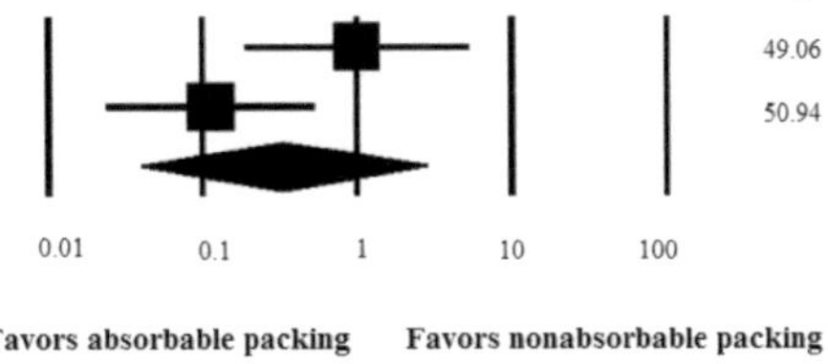

Figure 1. The odds ratios (OR) of postoperative synechia after FESS with absorbable vs. nonabsorbable nasal packing. Data are presented as OR with 95% confidence interval (CI). Heterogeneity test results: Q = 3.492, df = 1, P = 0.062, I2 = 71.37%.

Note that due to a significant between study heterogeneity, meta-analysis of the other postoperative outcomes was not possible.

4. Discussion

This is the first (to our knowledge) systematic review/meta-analysis to compare postoperative synechia efficacy and other outcomes of absorbable vs. nonabsorbable nasal packing after FESS for the treatment of chronic rhinosinusitis. A total of 241 nasal cavities in each treatment group within five randomized clinical trials met the inclusion criteria for this systematic review. The type of nasal packing material used among studies was considerably varied among other characteristics. Postoperative bleeding was less with absorbable packing, while postoperative pain and edema, pain and bleeding on packing removal found no between group differences or consistent findings. Our meta-analysis from the findings of two studies also revealed that when compared with nonabsorbable nasal packing, the incidence of postoperative synechia was not significantly reduced by absorbable nasal packing.

As noted earlier in our meta-analysis findings, the incidence of postoperative synechia for absorbable nasal packing was not significantly lower than nonabsorbable nasal packing. Among the studies in our systematic review, a markedly lower rate of synechia within

8 weeks of surgery among patients who received absorbable packing was reported by Szczygielski et al. [13]. Similarly, a non-eligible study (for the inclusion in our systematic review/meta-analysis), Hu et al. [16], reported that there was a reduced rate of postoperative synechia among patients who received absorbable nasal packing (Meropack) compared with those without packing. In contrary, little difference in the rate of postoperative synechia between patients who received absorbable (FloSeal) and nonabsorbable (Merocel) nasal packing was found in a prospective, non-randomized study by Baumann and Caversaccio [9]. Several other studies have also demonstrated no significant difference among packing with CMC, no packing, or nonabsorbable packing for reducing postoperative synechia [17, 18]. The lack of homogeneity was clearly shown by the disparate findings among studies, most notably in the type of absorbable packing material used. Due to this lack of homogeneity, we were restricted in our ability to make any definitive conclusions. However, the variability in synechia outcomes between studies does suggest that when it comes to reducing postoperative synechia, different types of absorbable packing materials are not created equal. Thus, in order to directly compare the efficacy of different absorbable packing materials for reducing synechia after FESS for the treatment of chronic rhinosinusitis, additional randomized trials are needed.

Although only two studies provided data on postoperative bleeding were included in our systematic review, both of these studies found decreased bleeding with absorbable packing. Several previous studies also suggest that packing with absorbable material (Meropack, Gelfoam) reduces postoperative bleeding compared with no packing [16, 19]. Jameson et al. [20] have also reported packing with absorbable material (FloSeal) decreased postoperative bleeding compared with nonabsorbable packing. In contrary, several other studies have found no difference in postoperative bleeding with absorbable (NasoPore, CMC) vs. nonabsorbable or no nasal packing [11, 21]. As with postoperative synechia, the disparate findings may be explained by the lack of homogeneity between studies. In order to further investigate the efficacy of absorbable vs. nonabsorbable nasal packing for preventing bleeding after FESS for treatment of chronic rhinosinusitis, additional randomized trials are needed.

We also examined other outcomes after FESS beside postoperative synechia and bleeding. These include postoperative edema and pain, and bleeding and pain on removal of packing. As expected, lack of consistency was again found in these results between studies. However, it should be mentioned that the study reported by Cho et al. [15], which had the most number of patients and according to our assessment, was the highest quality randomized controlled trial included, did reveal markedly less bleeding and pain on removal of absorbable nasal packing compared with nonabsorbable nasal packing.

A number of limitations must be mentioned in our study. One, both the type of packing material used and the duration of follow-up were different among the studies, which markedly restricted our ability to perform meta-analyses of the results. Two, our analyses did not take into account other important factors that may have biased the study findings, which consequently our meta-analysis, factors including indicators of packing efficacy, such as edema granulation and postoperative infection, associated pathologies, such as perioperative treatment, nasal polyps, postoperative debridement, aspirin sensitivity, smoking history, etc.

Three, we have decided not to include patient satisfaction as an outcome measure. Although when evaluating the effectiveness of any treatment, this is a very important consideration; we believe that it is more important to conclusively determine which means of nasal packing is most clinically effective. We do have to mention that the results from a previous randomized controlled trial, which was not eligible for inclusion in our systematic review/meta-analysis, suggested that the majority of patients prefer absorbable nasal packing material (specifically MeroGel) over nonabsorbable material [10]. Finally four, we only included a relatively small number of studies for our meta-analysis which limited the power of analysis. Lastly, due to the lack of data/sufficiently detailed methodological descriptions on the different types of FESS, we were not able to perform any analyses on them.

5. Conclusions

We were not able to make any definitive conclusions on the outcomes for the comparison of absorbable vs. nonabsorbable nasal packing material after FESS from the results of our systematic review and meta-analysis. Although there is some evidence to suggest that absorbable packing may be superior to nonabsorbable packing; lack of homogeneity between studies reported in the current literature, especially regarding the type of absorbable nasal packing material used, has become a major limiting factor for further analysis. Aside from the limiting factor, our systematic review also highlighted the fact that there is a limited amount of information available from high quality randomized trials on the efficacy of absorbable packing vs. nonabsorbable packing after FESS. In order to provide more definitive information on the absorbable packing vs. nonabsorbable packing and to compare the efficacy of different types of absorbable packing materials, additional randomized controlled trials are required. We hope such trials can be spurred by this study.

Acknowledgements

This study is supported in part by Taiwan Ministry of Health and Welfare Clinical Trial Center (MOHW105-TDU-B-212-133019).

Author details

Tang-Chuan Wang[1]* and Hung-Ta Hsiao[2]

*Address all correspondence to: tangchuan1020@gmail.com

1 Department of Otolaryngology—Head and Neck Surgery, China Medical University Hospital, Taiwan

2 Soteria Biotech Co. Ltd., National Tsing Hua University, Taiwan

References

[1] Benninger MS, Ferguson BJ, Hadley JA, Hamilos DL, Jacobs M, Kennedy DW, Lanza DC, Marple BF, Osguthorpe JD, Stankiewicz JA, Anon J, Denneny J, Emanuel I, Levine H. Adult chronic rhinosinusitis: Definitions, diagnosis, epidemiology, and pathophysiology. Otolaryngology–Head and Neck Surgery. 2003;**129**: S1–S32

[2] Welch KC, Stankiewicz JA. A contemporary review of endoscopic sinus surgery: techniques, tools, and outcomes. Laryngoscope, 2009;**119**:2258-2268

[3] Khalid AN, Quraishi SA, Kennedy DW. Long-term quality of life measures after functional endoscopic sinus surgery. American Journal of Rhinology. 2004;**18**:131-136

[4] Govindaraj S, Adappa ND, Kennedy DW. Endoscopic sinus surgery: Evolution and technical innovations. The Journal of Laryngology & Otology. 2010;**124**:242-250

[5] Palmer O, Moche JA, Matthews S. Endoscopic surgery of the nose and paranasal sinus. Oral & Maxillofacial Surgery Clinics of North America. 2012;**24**:275-283, ix

[6] Soler ZM, Mace J, Smith TL. Symptom-based presentation of chronic rhinosinusitis and symptom-specific outcomes after endoscopic sinus surgery. American Journal of Rhinology. 2008;**22**:297-301

[7] Tan BK, Chandra RK. Postoperative prevention and treatment of complications after sinus surgery. Otolaryngologic Clinics of North America. 2010;**43**:769-779

[8] Miller RS, Steward DL, Tami TA, Sillars MJ, Seiden AM, Shete M, Paskowski C, Welge J. The clinical effects of hyaluronic acid ester nasal dressing (Merogel) on intranasal wound healing after functional endoscopic sinus surgery. Otolaryngology–Head and Neck Surgery. 2003;**128**:862-869

[9] Baumann A, Caversaccio M. Hemostasis in endoscopic sinus surgery using a specific gelatin-thrombin based agent (FloSeal). Rhinology. 2003;**41**:244-249

[10] Franklin JH, Wright ED. Randomized, controlled, study of absorbable nasal packing on outcomes of surgical treatment of rhinosinusitis with polyposis. American Journal of Rhinology. 2007;**21**:214-217

[11] Shoman N, Gheriani H, Flamer D, Javer A. Prospective, double-blind, randomized trial evaluating patient satisfaction, bleeding, and wound healing using biodegradable synthetic polyurethane foam (NasoPore) as a middle meatal spacer in functional endoscopic sinus surgery. Journal of Otolaryngology—Head & Neck Surgery. 2009;**38**:112-118

[12] Berlucchi M, Castelnuovo P, Vincenzi A, Morra B, Pasquini E. Endoscopic utcomes of resorbable nasal packing after functional endoscopic sinus surgery: a multicenter prospective randomized controlled study. European Archives of Oto-Rhino-Laryngology. 2009;**266**:839-845

[13] Szczygielski K, Rapiejko P, Wojdas A, Jurkiewicz D. Use of CMC foam sinus dressing in FESS. European Archives of Oto-Rhino-Laryngology. 2010;**267**:537-540

[14] Wormald PJ, Boustred RN, Le T, Hawke L, Sacks R. A prospective single-blind randomized controlled study of use of hyaluronic acid nasal packs in patients after endoscopic sinus surgery. American Journal of Rhinology. 2006;**20**:7-10

[15] Cho KS, Shin SK, Lee JH, Kim JY, Koo SK, Kim YW, Kim MJ, Roh HJ. The efficacy of Cutanplast nasal packing after endoscopic sinus surgery: A prospective, randomized, controlled trial. Laryngoscope. 2013;**123**:564-568

[16] Hu KH, Lin KN, Li WT, Huang HM. Effects of Meropack in the middle meatus after functional endoscopic sinus surgery in children with chronic sinusitis. International Journal of Pediatric Otorhinolaryngology. 2008;**72**:1535-1540

[17] Leunig A, Betz CS, Siedek V, Kastl KG. CMC packing in functional endoscopic sinus surgery: Does it affect patient comfort? Rhinology. 2009;**47**:36-40

[18] Kastl KG, Betz CS, Siedek V, Leunig A. Effect of carboxymethylcellulose nasal packing on wound healing after functional endoscopic sinus surgery. American Journal of Rhinology & Allergy. 2009;**23**:80-84

[19] Wee JH, Lee CH, Rhee CS, Kim JW (2012) Comparison between Gelfoam packing and no packing after endoscopic sinus surgery in the same patients. European Archives of Oto-Rhino-Laryngology. 2012;**269**:897-903

[20] Jameson M, Gross CW, Kountakis SE. FloSeal use in endoscopic sinus surgery: effect on postoperative bleeding and synechiae formation. American Journal of Otolaryngology. 2006;**27**:86-90

[21] Kastl KG, Betz CS, Siedek V, Leunig A. Control of bleeding following functional endoscopic sinus surgery using carboxy-methylated cellulose packing. European Archives of Oto-Rhino-Laryngology. 2009;**266**:1239-1243

Section 5

Surgical Training

Chapter 5

The Role of Simulation in Endoscopic Sinus Surgery Training

Benjamin Stew and Eng Ooi

Additional information is available at the end of the chapter

http://dx.doi.org/10.5772/intechopen.69108

Abstract

Surgical simulation is an effective tool used to teach many of the fundamental skills required to be a surgeon. Simulation-based education with directed practice in surgical training allows repeated practice in an environment to learn surgical skills, which do not cause harm to patients. There are several simulators developed for endoscopic sinus surgery training. Some simulators have undergone validation studies with regard to developing skills necessary to perform endoscopic sinus surgery. This book chapter will review the currently available sinus surgery simulators that have undergone validation and evaluate their potential role in surgical training.

Keywords: simulation, sinus, surgery, training

1. Introduction

Rhinology and endoscopic sinus surgery (ESS) have advanced considerably over the last two decades owing to advances in technology and research. Accessing the skull base can now be achieved via a transnasal endoscopic approach, and our ability to deal with complex pathology has evolved given the dramatic improvement in our understanding of anatomy and development of new surgical instrumentation. However, there remains a need to achieve competency with basic ESS, which includes control of an endoscope as well as using instruments within the tight confines of the para-nasal sinuses close to vital structures such as the orbit or skull base. ESS requires familiarisation with the fulcrum effect of the instruments and the psychomotor constraints of the endoscopic interface. Resident participation in the operating room is associated with lengthier operative times [1, 2] and increased complication rates in ESS [3, 4]. Hence, there is a need for sinus surgery simulators to allow surgical training of residents in a safe environment thereby reducing complications. This chapter provides an updated review of ESS simulators and describes how simulation can be used effectively to improve training.

2. Brief overview of endoscopic sinus surgery

ESS is indicated in patients with chronic rhinosinusitis who fail to respond to medical therapy [5]. Minor complication rates are reportedly 5%, with postoperative epistaxis the most common. Major complication rates are less than 1%; however, these include orbital and carotid artery injuries, which are potentially devastating for the patient [6]. ESS is also now being extended to include the management of dysthyroid eye disease and epiphora [7, 8], and the surgical management of benign [9, 10] and malignant [11] sinonasal and skull base tumours.

3. Surgical training

Traditionally surgical training required trainees to undergo a 'surgical apprenticeship' where they would work long hours and perform a large number of cases in order to gain competency. However, surgical competency does not always correlate with the number of cases performed. Critical to the achievement of expertise is the number of hours spent in deliberate practice [12]. Most developed countries advocate for safe working hours which is usually to restrict the working hours of residents/junior doctors in order to avoid fatigue and improve patient safety. There is therefore a need to provide trainees with the opportunity to undertake deliberate practice within the confines of these safe working hours. While traditional didactic teaching and textbooks remain of utmost importance, it has been demonstrated that the current generation of trainees is more amenable to technology and alternative teaching methods [13]. Interactive, hands-on experiences with the opportunity to learn through trial and error are considered more enjoyable and effective [14].

This evolution, with respect to surgical skills acquisition, requires a change in the traditional methods of training. It is not always possible or safe for a trainee to practise and acquire the surgical skills that were traditionally learned in the operating theatre during operations on patients. Alternatives such as watching live or recorded surgery and cadaveric dissection have become an essential part of the way in which training is delivered. Cadaveric dissection remains the gold standard of ESS training and forms part of the otolaryngology curriculum in many training programmes [15]. Factors, such as cost and cadaver availability, however, limit the amount of time and opportunity that a trainee may have to work on their skills at cadaveric courses.

In areas, outside of medicine where significant harm is associated with error, simulation has been successfully implemented. Industries, such as aviation, use simulation for the purpose of providing a safe environment for pilots to practise, which reduces training time through improved retention of information. Simulation in surgery is rapidly developing and becoming a popular way to train both novice and skilled doctors. Repetitive practice of a well-defined task and feedback allow for an accelerated and ultimately safer learning curve [16]. Simulation has the potential to improve surgical training including techniques and understanding, advances in instrumentation, patient safety and time allocation in theatre [3].

4. Simulation

Surgical simulators vary considerably and range from devices that can be used to teach simple skills through to more complicated techniques. **Table 1** summarises the different types of simulation models that exist as well as their advantages, disadvantages and best use.

Many sinus surgery simulators have been developed around the world varying from simple models constructed from regular household items to highly complex virtual reality models. Physical models described in the literature include low-cost, low-fidelity models through to high cost and intermediate fidelity ones. The major limitation of synthetic models is the unrealistic anatomy and consistency of the tissue, which lacks mobility and lifelike strength. Despite this, many have proven to be useful training tools for ESS trainees. Several studies have shown that the technical skills acquired on low-fidelity physical models might confer the same degree of benefit as high-fidelity training models, such as cadavers. This was because the learning process was considered to be more important than the physical substrate [18]. The Georgetown low-cost sinus trainer costs $5 and allows the trainee to practise basic endoscopy and sinus surgery skills including recess probing, targeted injections, removal of a suture, removal of a foreign body and antrostomy creation using an egg [19, 20]. Witterick's group from the

Simulation	Advantages	Disadvantages	Best use
Bench models	Cheap, portable, reusable, minimal risk	Low fidelity, basic tasks, tasks are not surgical operations	Basic skills for novice learners, discrete skills
Live animals	High fidelity, can practise haemostasis	High cost, ethical considerations, anatomical differences between animals and humans, single use only	Advanced practice of dissection skills
Cadavers	High fidelity, only 'true' anatomical simulator	High cost, limited availability, single use, tissue compliance different from live surgery, infection risk	Advanced procedural knowledge, practice of dissection skills
Human performance simulators	Reusable, high fidelity, data capture, interactivity	Cost, maintenance (upkeep), limited technical applications	Team training, crisis management
Virtual reality surgical simulators	Reusable, data capture, minimal setup time, photorealism, potential for haptic feedback	Moderate to high cost, maintenance (upkeep), acceptance by trainees	Basic and advanced endoscopic sinus surgery

Table 1. Types of surgical simulators available [17].

University of Toronto developed a low-cost, low-fidelity, easily constructed simulator for $20 with five different training modules and demonstrated that training on the model had a positive impact on ESS skills [21, 22]. More recently, the University of Texas [23] have produced a silicone injection moulded ESS simulation model at low cost and testing revealed high ratings for both face and construct validity. Storz have crafted a lifelike training model based on real computed tomography images. This can be purchased but is considerably more expensive than those already discussed and furthermore the model has not undergone adequate validation [24].

Live animal and cadaveric simulation offers trainees excellent handling fidelity. They also offer the advantage of possessing tissue realism including bleeding. Tissue realism is, however, variable, depending on whether the cadaver is embalmed or fresh frozen. Embalmed cadavers do not exhibit the same subtle tissue characteristics of fresh frozen tissue. Normal surgical instruments may be used on either, and recognised surgical procedures may be undertaken. Live animal simulation is not permitted in all countries including the UK, and therefore, cadaveric simulation is more common. ESS simulation on cadavers has many advantages over physical models, but it relies on cadaver availability [25, 26]. The most important advantage is that cadavers represent the only true anatomical model of the human para-nasal sinuses. Unfortunately, cost and ethical approval are two factors mitigating widespread practice. Cadaveric simulation also poses an infection risk and specimens are limited to single use. The ovine sinus simulator utilises a cadaveric sheep's head whose sinus configuration has some similarities to human anatomy, including the lateral position of the maxillary sinuses, posterosuperior position of the skull base and midline of the position of the septum. The sheep's head, however, is longer, lacks a sphenoid sinus and has poorly aerated ethmoidal cells rendering ethmoidectomy unrealistic [27].

Although early simulators were largely cadaveric or synthetic, technology advancement has resulted in a boom of virtual reality simulators. Virtual reality (VR) simulators have the capacity to overcome the inadequacies of physical and cadaveric models and allow trainees to practise a standardised, task with objective feedback. Sinus surgery naturally lends itself to computerised simulation given the use of high-definition screens and requirement of the operator to work from a 2D image for a 3D procedure [28]. One of the earliest VR simulators was the Madigan endoscopic sinus surgery simulator (ES3), a simulator developed in collaboration with Department of Defence contractor Lockheed Martin Corporation in 1996. The operating system allows for visual and haptic feedback, offers instruction and analyses performance. It facilitates ESS training through provision of spatial relationships and depiction of sinus anatomy, as well as allowing the trainee to use common surgical instruments and has three difficulty modes depending on ability. Other VR simulators have been described in the literature. However, only three other VR simulators have undergone validation studies (**Table 3**). The McGill simulator for ESS (MSESS), developed by the National Research Council of Canada, represents the most advanced VR ESS simulator that is currently available to purchase. It has the ability to simulate an ethmoidectomy and sphenoidotomy secondary to its high optical resolution and tissue removal algorithm. The performance metrics relating to quality, efficiency and safety demonstrated a dichotomy between novice and senior surgeons [29]. Widespread adoption of the MSESS in training may, however, prove unrealistic as a consequence of its cost.

The Flinders sinus surgery simulator (FSSS) is a prototype that was developed at Flinders University and was funded by The Garnett Passe and Rodney Williams Memorial Foundation. It is a high-resolution haptic simulator that has advanced photorealism but a relatively basic tissue removal algorithm and lacks realistic haptic feedback. Unfortunately it is not currently available for purchase and is not being used as part of a training programme. The Dextroscope is a commercial FDA approved simulator developed by volume interactions. It facilitates reconstruction of images from a patient's computed tomographic scan. The simulator uses virtual tools through stereoscopic glass; however, it lacks force feedback and is time consuming.

5. Validation

Validation refers to the process of testing the simulator, and it can be defined as outlined in **Table 2**.

Validation is an essential process prior to the implementation of a simulator into training. Face validation is simplest and is often undertaken first and refers to the simulator looking and feeling authentic. In the case of ESS simulation, it requires judgement from a person familiar with ESS, which is typically an expert rhinologist. In isolation, it is never sufficient and requires further evaluation before acceptable conclusions, regarding its ability to teach and train, are able to drawn. It is fundamental that a surgical simulator undergoes construct validation. Construct validity refers to the assessment of the quality of the simulator and its ability to carry out what it was designed to do. This may be the teaching of anatomy or ESS skills and should have the ability to distinguish novices from experts. Fundamentally, the goal of surgical simulation is to improve surgical performance and efficiency. Predictive validity represents the highest level of testing. A sinus simulator that has undergone predictive validation has the ability to teach those skills that can be translated into improved operative performance.

There are seven physical trainers, one cadaveric model and four VR platforms that have undergone validation as ESS simulators (**Table 3**).

5.1. Physical bench models

There are a number of physical bench models that have undergone validation in the literature. All seven of these models score well with respect to teaching endoscopy skills and hand eye coordination. Efficiency of task completion improved with practice. Camera navigation and instrument handling became more accurate. These observations were particularly apparent among medical students and resident learners. While these models lend themselves to these basic tasks, their use as a training tool for ESS would appear limited. They do not aid surgical decision-making nor have the realism to teach surgical anatomy. The low-fidelity sinus simulator developed by the University of Toronto was, however, able to demonstrate that its use prior to cadaveric dissection improved surgical performance. Given the ease of construction, low cost and overall entertainment factor, these low-fidelity physical models may be implemented into training to teach novices and junior trainee's simple skills in ESS.

	Definition	Use
Face	Having experts review the contents of the test to see if it measures what it is supposed to measure	To initially design a test (subjective)
Content	An estimate of the validity of a testing instrument based on a detailed examination of the contents of the test item	Experts review whether or not the test contains the logical steps and skill used in a procedure (subjective)
Construct	A set of procedures for evaluating a testing instrument based on the degree to which the test items identify the quality, ability, or trait it was designed to measure	To differentiate between novices and experts (objective)
Predictive	The extent to which the scores on a test are predictive of actual performance	Test used to measure skill predicts who will actually perform the procedure well and who will not in the operating room. This provides the most clinically useful assessment (objective)

Table 2. Validity definitions—reproduced from Ref. [16].

5.2. Cadaveric/ovine models

Cadaveric simulation, despite being regarded as the gold standard over physical and VR models, is yet to demonstrate that its use improves operating performance. Nonetheless trainees do consider the experience of training on cadavers to be highly valuable [15]. The sheep's head model as a sinus simulator for the purpose of ESS training has undergone face and construct validation [27, 45]. Awad et al. suggest that it used as a step in the simulation ladder, prior to in-vivo practice, as it represents an opportunity to focus on basic endoscopic rhinological procedures in conjunction with training on VR and cadaveric models. They describe a task specific checklist and global assessment tool to evaluate the performance of the operator. The simulator demonstrated a clear relationship between surgical experience and task performance.

5.3. Virtual reality models

The most comprehensively validated VR sinus simulator is the ES3. The ES3 has undergone extensive validation and to date represents the only VR ESS simulator to have predictive validity. It has been shown to train novices in sinus surgery, so that they can perform to a level within 80% of an experienced surgeon. Surgical performance within the operating theatre, as judged anonymously by senior surgeons, was better following simulation training. The positive impact of prior simulation training was reflected in the fact that surgeons reported improvement in confidence and observed reduced overall operating time. The ES3, however, is not currently available to purchase for residency training programmes. The MSESS has also been systematically validated and research shows that it is able to differentiate between levels of experience based on task performance. Violation of no-go zones and the amount of mucosa resected over the lamina papyracea were both significantly higher in novices. The simulator demonstrates adequate realism and serves as a useful training option for medical students through to senior surgeons. The FSSS is a prototype that is currently not available for purchase

Simulator	Analysis	Validity
Physical bench model		
• SIMONT	Stamm et al. [30]	Face
• Storz Sinus model	Fortes et al. [31]	Face
• Oklahoma FESS model	Briner et al. [24]	Face
• Georgetown Sinus trainer	Burge et al. [32]	Construct
• Toronto Sinus simulator	Steehler et al. [20]	Face, content & construct
• Texas ESS model	Steehler et al. [33]	Construct*
• Seattle Sinus task trainer	Leung et al. [21]	Predictive
	Wais et al. [22]	Face
	Chang et al. [23]	Face, content & construct
	Harbison et al. [2]	
Cadaveric/ovine		
Sheep's head model	Awad et al. [27]	Face, content & construct
	Awad et al. [34]	
Virtual reality		
• Madigan (ES3)	Rudman et al. [35]	Face
• McGill (MSESS)	Edmond et al. [36]	Predictive
• Flinders (FSSS)	Uribe et al. [37]	Face & construct
• Dextroscope	Arora et al. [38]	Construct
	Fried at al. [39]	Construct
	Solyar et al. [40]	Construct
	Fried et al. [41]	Predictive
	Varshney et al. [29]	Face & construct
	Dharmawardana et al. [42]	Face & content
	Diment et al. [43]	Construct
	Caversaccio et al. [44]	Predictive*

*Unable to prove.

Table 3. Summary of validated sinus surgery simulators.

and it is not incorporated in a training programme. As a simulator, it was considered better among novices compared to experts in terms of usability and usefulness. While tissue texture and deformity was considered realistic, the haptic behaviour of the rigid endoscope was not. Task performance was significantly different between novices and experts demonstrating construct validity for the FSSS. The Dextroscope failed to demonstrate a significant improvement in a trainees' anatomical knowledge following its use and lacks any proven validity.

5.4. Limitations

There have been numerous publications describing the validation of sinus simulators that now exist but like many other specialties, interpreting the accuracy of these studies can be problematic [46]. Typically, authors describe simulators that have been evaluated with a view to validation. However, the quality of the study, outcome measures and statistical analysis lack accuracy and clarity rendering the conclusions weak. Statements of effectiveness and representativeness by an expert in the field do not constitute high-level evidence. Face validity relies on expert opinion but unfortunately no universal consensus exists as to what constitutes an expert. Furthermore, novices are poorly categorised and range from students to middle tier trainees. Several of the above studies, while well constructed, involve low sample sizes and therefore lack the power to make valid conclusions. This lack of standardisation in terms of recruitment and outcome reporting make it very difficult to compare one simulator with another. Therefore, choosing one simulator over another is difficult. Aside from the limitations that exist in terms of validation, simulators are expensive and require frequent maintenance.

6. The future of simulation

The role of simulation in surgical training is already well established. Simulation serves to improve the technical skills required of a surgeon within both otolaryngology and other surgical subspecialties [47, 48]. The widespread implementation of simulation in training is influenced by many factors such as cost and effectiveness. The provision of simulation opportunities for surgical trainees depends on departmental and training programme philosophy, pre-existing access to cadaveric workshops and courses, and ultimately a need to change practice. Undoubtedly, high-fidelity models will become increasingly available and cost effective and allow departments to utilise simulation for assessment of surgical skills acquired rather than as a training tool. This may be as part of trainee assessment and recruitment or revalidation. Competency, which currently relies upon expert opinion or logbook analysis, may be superseded by simulation. Laeeq et al. [49] demonstrated that a minimum of 55 sinus surgeries are required to achieve competency in all steps of FESS; however, training requires formative and summative assessment and not simply operative cases only. Procedural-based assessments, which are routinely used in many training programmes for assessment, are subject to the inherent bias of the well-liked trainee scoring highly. Objective structured assessment of skills (OSATS) have been developed and shown to be effective in the assessment of surgical competence [33]. Their application to a simulation task that has the potential to be blinded and independently reviewed is an exciting possibility. Alternatively training departments could use the objective scores that are given by simulators for score specific tasks.

7. Key points

- Simulation provides trainees of all abilities an opportunity to improve their skills in a safe, low-risk environment

- ESS simulators exist with inherent advantages and disadvantages
- Simulation can be used to practise simple and complex skills
- Validation is a fundamental aspect of simulation development
- Simulation has a key role to play in the evolution of surgical training

Author details

Benjamin Stew[1]* and Eng Ooi[2]

*Address all correspondence to: stewb@doctors.org.uk

1 Flinders Medical Centre, Adelaide, Australia

2 Flinders Medical Centre, Flinders University, Adelaide, Australia

References

[1] Dedhia RC, Lord CA, Pinheiro-Neto CD, Fernandez-Miranda JC, Wang EW, Gardner PA, et al. Endoscopic endonasal pituitary surgery: Impact of surgical education on operation length and patient morbidity. Journal of Neurological Surgery Part B: Skull Base. 2012;**73**(6):405–409

[2] Harbison RA, Johnson KE, Miller C, Sardesai MG, Davis GE. Face, content, and construct validation of a low-cost, non-biologic, sinus surgery task trainer and knowledge-based curriculum. International Forum of Allergy & Rhinology. 2016;**7**

[3] Gross RD, Sheridan MF, Burgess LP. Endoscopic sinus surgery complications in residency. The Laryngoscope. 1997;**107**(8):1080–1085

[4] Kinsella JB, Calhoun KH, Bradfield JJ, Hokanson JA, Bailey BJ. Complications of endoscopic sinus surgery in a residency training program. The Laryngoscope. 1995;**105**(10):1029–1032

[5] Dautremont JF, Rudmik L. When are we operating for chronic rhinosinusitis? A systematic review of maximal medical therapy protocols prior to endoscopic sinus surgery. International Forum of Allergy & Rhinology. 2015;**5**(12):1095–1103

[6] Ramakrishnan VR, Kingdom TT, Nayak JV, Hwang PH, Orlandi RR. Nationwide incidence of major complications in endoscopic sinus surgery. International Forum of Allergy & Rhinology. 2012;**2**(1):34–39

[7] Leong SC, Karkos PD, Macewen CJ, White PS. A systematic review of outcomes following surgical decompression for dysthyroid orbitopathy. The Laryngoscope. 2009;**119**(6):1106–1115

[8] Leong SC, Macewen CJ, White PS. A systematic review of outcomes after dacryocystorhinostomy in adults. American Journal of Rhinology & Allergy. 2010;**24**(1):81–90

[9] Wormald PJ, Ooi E, van Hasselt CA, Nair S. Endoscopic removal of sinonasal inverted papilloma including endoscopic medial maxillectomy. The Laryngoscope. 2003;**113**(5):867–873

[10] Robinson S, Patel N, Wormald PJ. Endoscopic management of benign tumors extending into the infratemporal fossa: A two-surgeon transnasal approach. The Laryngoscope. 2005;**115**(10):1818–1822

[11] Jardeleza C, Seiberling K, Floreani S, Wormald PJ. Surgical outcomes of endoscopic management of adenocarcinoma of the sinonasal cavity. Rhinology. 2009;**47**(4):354–361

[12] Fried GM, Feldman LS. Objective assessment of technical performance. World Journal of Surgery. 2008;**32**(2):156–160

[13] Glaser AY, Hall CB, Uribe SJ, Fried MP. Medical students' attitudes toward the use of an endoscopic sinus surgery simulator as a training tool. American Journal of Rhinology. 2006;**20**(2):177–179

[14] Mangold K. Educating a new generation: Teaching baby boomer faculty about millennial students. Nurse Educator. 2007;**32**(1):21–23

[15] Anastakis DJ, Regehr G, Reznick RK, Cusimano M, Murnaghan J, Brown M, et al. Assessment of technical skills transfer from the bench training model to the human model. American Journal of Surgery. 1999;**177**(2):167–170

[16] Reznick RK, MacRae H. Teaching surgical skills—changes in the wind. The New England Journal of Medicine. 2006;**355**(25):2664–2669

[17] Ooi EH, Witterick IJ. Rhinologic surgical training. Otolaryngologic Clinics of North America. 2010;**43**(3):673–689

[18] Hamstra SJ, Dubrowski A, Backstein D. Teaching technical skills to surgical residents: A survey of empirical research. Clinical Orthopaedics and Related Research. 2006;**449**:108–115

[19] Malekzadeh S, Pfisterer MJ, Wilson B, Na H, Steehler MK. A novel low-cost sinus surgery task trainer. Otolaryngology—Head and Neck Surgery. 2011;**145**(4):530–533

[20] Steehler MK, Pfisterer MJ, Na H, Hesham HN, Pehlivanova M, Malekzadeh S. Face, content, and construct validity of a low-cost sinus surgery task trainer. Otolaryngology—Head and Neck Surgery. 2012;**146**(3):504–509

[21] Leung RM, Leung J, Vescan A, Dubrowski A, Witterick I. Construct validation of a low-fidelity endoscopic sinus surgery simulator. American Journal of Rhinology. 2008;**22**(6):642–648

[22] Wais M, Ooi E, Leung RM, Vescan AD, Lee J, Witterick IJ. The effect of low-fidelity endoscopic sinus surgery simulators on surgical skill. International Forum of Allergy & Rhinology. 2012;**2**(1):20–26

[23] Chang DR, Lin RP, Bowe S, Bunegin L, Weitzel EK, McMains KC, et al. Fabrication and validation of a low-cost, medium-fidelity silicone injection molded endoscopic sinus surgery simulation model. The Laryngoscope. 2016;**127**

[24] Briner HR, Simmen D, Jones N, Manestar D, Manestar M, Lang A, et al. Evaluation of an anatomic model of the paranasal sinuses for endonasal surgical training. Rhinology. 2007;**45**(1):20–23

[25] Mills R, Lee P. Surgical skills training in middle-ear surgery. The Journal of Laryngology and Otology. 2003;**117**(3):159–163

[26] McCarthy MC, Ranzinger MR, Nolan DJ, Lambert CS, Castillo MH. Accuracy of cricothyroidotomy performed in canine and human cadaver models during surgical skills training. Journal of the American College of Surgeons. 2002;**195**(5):627–629

[27] Awad Z, Touska P, Arora A, Ziprin P, Darzi A, Tolley NS. Face and content validity of sheep heads in endoscopic rhinology training. International Forum of Allergy & Rhinology. 2014;**4**(10):851–858

[28] Ecke U, Klimek L, Muller W, Ziegler R, Mann W. Virtual reality: Preparation and execution of sinus surgery. Computer Aided Surgery. 1998;**3**(1):45–50

[29] Varshney R, Frenkiel S, Nguyen LH, Young M, Del Maestro R, Zeitouni A, et al. The McGill simulator for endoscopic sinus surgery (MSESS): A validation study. Journal of Otolaryngology—Head & Neck Surgery. 2014;**43**:40

[30] Stamm A, Nogueira JF, Lyra M. Feasibility of balloon dilatation in endoscopic sinus surgery simulator. Otolaryngology—Head and Neck Surgery. 2009;**140**(3):320–323

[31] Fortes B, Balsalobre L, Weber R, Stamm R, Stamm A, Oto F, et al. Endoscopic sinus surgery dissection courses using a real simulator: The benefits of this training. Brazilian Journal of Otorhinolaryngology. 2016;**82**(1):26–32

[32] Burge SD, Bunegin L, Weitzel EK, McMains KC. The validation of an endoscopic sinus surgery skills training model: A pilot study. American Journal of Rhinology & Allergy. 2012;**26**(5):409–413

[33] Steehler MK, Chu EE, Na H, Pfisterer MJ, Hesham HN, Malekzadeh S. Teaching and assessing endoscopic sinus surgery skills on a validated low-cost task trainer. The Laryngoscope. 2013;**123**(4):841–844

[34] Awad Z, Taghi A, Sethukumar P, Tolley NS. Construct validity of the ovine model in endoscopic sinus surgery training. The Laryngoscope. 2015;**125**(3):539–543

[35] Rudman DT, Stredney D, Sessanna D, Yagel R, Crawfis R, Heskamp D, et al. Functional endoscopic sinus surgery training simulator. The Laryngoscope. 1998;**108**(11 Pt 1):1643–1647

[36] Edmond CV Jr. Impact of the endoscopic sinus surgical simulator on operating room performance. The Laryngoscope. 2002;**112**(7 I):1148–1158

[37] Uribe JI, Ralph WM Jr, Glaser AY, Fried MP. Learning curves, acquisition, and retention of skills trained with the endoscopic sinus surgery simulator. American Journal of Rhinology. 2004;**18**(2):87–92

[38] Arora H, Uribe J, Ralph W, Zeltsan M, Cuellar H, Gallagher A, et al. Assessment of construct validity of the endoscopic sinus surgery simulator. Archives of Otolaryngology—Head & Neck Surgery. 2005;**131**(3):217–221

[39] Fried MP, Sadoughi B, Weghorst SJ, Zeltsan M, Cuellar H, Uribe JI, et al. Construct validity of the endoscopic sinus surgery simulator: II. Assessment of discriminant validity and expert benchmarking. Archives of Otolaryngology—Head & Neck Surgery. 2007;**133**(4):350–357

[40] Solyar A, Cuellar H, Sadoughi B, Olson TR, Fried MP. Endoscopic sinus surgery simulator as a teaching tool for anatomy education. American Journal of Surgery. 2008;**196**(1):120–124

[41] Fried MP, Sadoughi B, Gibber MJ, Jacobs JB, Lebowitz RA, Ross DA, et al. From virtual reality to the operating room: The endoscopic sinus surgery simulator experiment. Otolaryngology—Head and Neck Surgery. 2010;**142**(2):202–207

[42] Dharmawardana N, Ruthenbeck G, Woods C, Elmiyeh B, Diment L, Ooi EH, et al. Validation of virtual-reality-based simulations for endoscopic sinus surgery. Clinical Otolaryngology. 2015;**40**(6):569–579

[43] Diment LE, Ruthenbeck GS, Dharmawardana N, Carney AS, Woods CM, Ooi EH, et al. Comparing surgical experience with performance on a sinus surgery simulator. ANZ Journal of Surgery. 2016;**86**(12):990–995

[44] Caversaccio M, Eichenberger A, Häusler R. Virtual simulator as a training tool for endonasal surgery. American Journal of Rhinology. 2003;**17**(5):283–290

[45] Delgado-Vargas B, Romero-Salazar AL, Reyes Burneo PM, Vasquez Hincapie C, de Los Santos Granado G, Del Castillo Lopez R, et al. Evaluation of resident's training for endoscopic sinus surgery using a sheep's head. European Archives of Oto-Rhino-Laryngology. 2016;**273**(8):2085–2089

[46] Schout BM, Hendrikx AJ, Scherpbier AJ, Bemelmans BL. Update on training models in endourology: A qualitative systematic review of the literature between January 1980 and April 2008. European Urology. 2008;**54**(6):1247–1261

[47] Fitzgerald TN, Duffy AJ, Bell RL, Berman L, Longo WE, Roberts KE. Computer-based endoscopy simulation: Emerging roles in teaching and professional skills assessment. Journal of Surgical Education. 2008;**65**(3):229–235

[48] Verdaasdonk EG, Dankelman J, Lange JF, Stassen LP. Transfer validity of laparoscopic knot-tying training on a VR simulator to a realistic environment: A randomized controlled trial. Surgical Endoscopy. 2008;**22**(7):1636–1642

[49] Laeeq K, Lin SY, Varela DA, Lane AP, Reh D, Bhatti NI. Achievement of competency in endoscopic sinus surgery of otolaryngology residents. The Laryngoscope. 2013;**123**(12):2932–2934